STRE

MANAGEMENT

Simple Ways to Manage Stress Find Lasting Peace of Mind

(Guided Meditation Techniques to Eliminate Stress)

Joyce Mills

Published by Tomas Edwards

© **Joyce Mills**

All Rights Reserved

Stress Management: Simple Ways to Manage Stress Find Lasting Peace of Mind (Guided Meditation Techniques to Eliminate Stress)

ISBN 978-1-990268-27-4

Legal & Disclaimer

The information contained in this book is not designed to replace or take the place of any form of medicine or professional medical advice. The information in this book has been provided for educational and entertainment purposes only.

The information contained in this book has been compiled from sources deemed reliable, and it is accurate to the best of the Author's knowledge; however, the Author cannot guarantee its accuracy and validity and cannot be held liable for any errors or omissions. Changes are periodically made to this book. You must consult your doctor or get professional medical advice before using any of the suggested remedies, techniques, or information in this book.

Upon using the information contained in this book, you agree to hold harmless the Author from and against any damages, costs, and expenses, including any legal fees potentially resulting from the application of any of the information provided by this guide. This disclaimer applies to any damages or injury caused by the use and application, whether directly or indirectly, of any advice or information presented, whether for breach of contract, tort, negligence, personal injury, criminal intent, or under any other cause of action.

You agree to accept all risks of using the information presented inside this book. You need to consult a professional medical practitioner in order to ensure you are both able and healthy enough to participate in this program.

Table of Contents

Introduction

He has conducted many years of research interviews with outstandingly successful, highly effective men and women, from all walks of life. These top achievers have included scientists, inventors, authors, explorers, sporting world champions and millionaire entrepreneurs. During these interviews, these people shared the secrets of their personal effectiveness, their thought and behaviour systems and processes enabling us to better understand how they are seemingly more stress free than the rest of us, and perhaps more importantly therefore, understand how we can become more effective ourselves.

We can gain an insight into the ways they think and behave, so that we can do the same and hopefully have more energy, time and less stress along the way.

These research interviews shed light onto the ways in which these people actually prevent stress rather than manage it. After all, why would you want to manage stress if you could prevent it?

Chapter 1: Adopting The Right Work Habits

We have just talked about work being one of the biggest sources of stress. I am not implying that you should stop working because of this. That would be unreasonable. The problem is, more than likely, you have poor working habits that result in more stress.

So, your first step in handling stress is by looking at how you can adopt the right work habits.

Let's look at some of the ways you can do that.

1: Keep Busy

It may come as a shock to you to find that keeping busy can help you relieve stress. But trust me, it works.

It works because it keeps you from staying idle.

The thing is, stress tends to kick in when you are idle. When you are idle, all kinds of thoughts flood your mind. These thoughts have the ability to make you anxious or even stress out about a number of things, most of which center around the uncertainty of the future and some regrets of the past.

So, in order to avoid this, you have to get busy doing work that is mentally engaging. And since your mind cannot focus on two things at the same time, you will effectively combat stress.

I am not making this up by the way. Research by the University of Chicago in collaboration with Shanghai Jiao Tong University established that people who stay busy all day tend to be happier than those who aren't.

Let's look at another technique.

2: Rest While At Work

Fatigue is one of the signs that show that you are stressed.

At the same time, your body is more likely to be stressed when you are tired. A little bit of rest can go a long way in keeping you from getting tired and in this way keep you from getting stressed.

Getting some time during the day to get some rest can help lower your fatigue, and by doing so, you can reduce you stress levels or even prevent stress from attacking and overwhelming you.

My opinion? No.

That is what research from the Endocrine Society, which was published in Medical Daily revealed. According to the researchers, even a 30 minute nap during the day can help reverse the effects of poor sleep during the night, reduce your stress and give you an immunity boost.

Personally, I get a nap 30 minutes after lunch and this keeps me going for more than 12 hours of work in a day.

Does this sound like good enough for you? If so, go ahead and adjust your life accordingly.

3: Relax As You Do Your Work

Another thing that you can do to keep stress at bay is learning to stay calm as you work.

There is this notion in society that makes it seem like you will get better at your job by straining. However, the truth is that straining doesn't make you better and it isn't necessary.

Straining only makes it more likely that you will become anxious and consequently stressed. In fact, Anxiety Center has found a very close relationship between stress and muscle strain.

To stop strain at work from making you stressed, simply remember to keep calm while at work, and you will have less stress. Do not make your work harder than it needs to be.

4: Practice Effective Time Management

Being able to manage your time well can greatly help reduce stress.

Most of us deal with many tasks in a typical day. Sometimes when you look at the list of items in your daily to-do list, you may feel some anxiety creeping in.

If you want to avoid that anxiety, it is necessary that you go through your list and prioritize the activities in it then arrange them in their order of importance. Also, set aside time for your hobbies and things that bring you joy. Once you do that, you will find that you have more time to do the things that truly matter.

You will also realize that the consequence of not dealing with the unimportant tasks is something that you can easily live with. And by doing this, your stress levels will go down and you will live a better life.

5: Do One Thing At A Time

When you wake up in the morning, it may sometimes feel like there are a hundred tasks that need to be accomplished.

This realization can make you stressed. We have already seen that creating a prioritized to-do list can help you to handle things in a much better way and relieves some of your stress.

But, it doesn't stop there.

You also need the discipline to take on the tasks, one at a time. You need to trust your plan and follow it accordingly without mixing things up.

Think of an hour-glass. Only one grain of sand can pass through the neck of the glass. Not two, not three, but just one. You have to adopt the same mantra.

One task at a time, one grain of sand at a time, and you will get through the day safely with less stress. Go ahead, give it a try.

6: Take Time Off When Ill

You may make the mistake of working when you are ill. However, doing so only makes you more stressed and worsens your bottom-line.

This is especially true if you work at a job that puts you under pressure. The Harvard business review reports that if your work in high-pressure jobs, your stress situation gets worse.

During times of stress, your brain stimulates the production of hormones that increase your heart rate, blood pressure and make your muscles tense. However, what you need to know is that your body cannot maintain this state for long and it begins to break down in various ways, often with serious consequences such as headaches, insomnia, heart attacks, hypertension, stroke and the like.

So, to avoid such eventualities, if you are ill, take some time off and allow your body to repair itself. Engaging in constant work even when you are unwell is a recipe for disaster.

7: Get Enough Sleep

One of the many reasons why you may be stressed is because you may not be getting enough sleep. WebMD reports that when you do not get enough sleep, your body produces more of the hormone cortisol. Cortisol is one of the main stress hormones in the body. So, if you are not getting enough sleep, you are only making your stress problems worse.

You need to reschedule your program such that it allows you to get around 7 to 8 hours of sleep. The problem however is that sometimes you may be setting aside enough time for sleep, but your stress keeps you from getting quality sleep.

If this is what happens to you, there are some things you could do to make yourself get better sleep:

Make sure that your bedroom is a calm place and one that has little (if any) distractions.

Avoid taking caffeine just before you get to bed. Caffeine is meant to promote alertness and this may affect your sleep.

Avoid working on mentally exhausting tasks before you get to bed, so that your mind gets enough time to relax and calm down.

Try getting a hot bath and reading a book that isn't mentally exhausting.

Try making some sleep adjustments to your current way of life and things may start getting better.

Now that we have looked at some of the ways you can change our working habits, let us look at another way you can fight stress...

Chapter 2: Symptoms Of Stress

How do you know if the stress you are experiencing is harmful or beneficial? There are some key signs that accompany each type of stress. Positive stress (or "eustress") tends to be more short-term than long-term and has more positive effects on your mental and physical well-being. It motivates, excites, and boosts your performance. You tend to view it as something within your control and abilities to successfully deal with.

Negative stress (or "distress"), on the other hand, can be short or long-term. It can trigger general symptoms of anxiety, discomfort, and decreases performance. It can hamper your immune system, trigger insomnia and/or depression, and can dampen your energy level. Whereas positive stress is usually seen as something within your control and in your skillset, negative stress is usually seen as something outside of your control and capability to handle.

Some common signs of short-term stress include:

-Dry   mouth
-Increased   heart   rate
-Rapid   breathing
-Muscle   spasms
-Headaches
-Increased   bathroom   visits
-Shortness   of   breath
-General   lethargy   and   fatigue
-Increased   sweat   production
-Tense   muscles
-Cold   hands,   feet,   and   skin
-A nauseous "butterflies" feeling in your stomach

If short-term stress symptoms are not recognized or dealt with in a healthy way, they may morph into long-term stress conditions.

Long-term stress can manifest itself in the following   symptoms:
-Persistent moods of frustration, anger, or

anxiety
-Reduced   enjoyment   in   life
-Distractibility
-Hampered   decision   making
-Making   bad   choices
-A tendency to view challenges as
threatening   and   overpowering
-Feelings   of   rejection
-Unwillingness to discuss personal
problems   with   friends   or   family
-Inability   to   work
-Fear   of   free   time
- A hampered ability to laugh
-Constantly feeling tired, even after
getting   a   good   night's   sleep

What is Anxiety?

According to the Anxiety and Depression
Association of America, anxiety affects
18% of adults in America alone. An
individual with anxiety is three to five
times more likely to visit a doctor and six
times more likely to be hospitalized in a
psych ward than the average person.
About 1/3 of the U.S.'s health fund goes

towards helping those with anxiety disorders.

Although anxiety can be caused by a variety of factors, stress is a major factor that fuels anxiety. The Mayo Clinic supports this theory, citing examples of stress buildup or stress due to an illness. Stress buildup happens during an accumulation of smaller stressors in your life like financial problems, relational conflicts, or traffic. Stress due to having an illness or having a family member with an illness can trigger worry about the future and can cause anxiety.

Anxiety is an excessive feeling of worry, nervousness, apprehension, and dread. It can vary in intensity. Mild anxiety usually causes a feeling of uneasiness and apprehension. Severe anxiety can hamper one's ability to function, sleep, or work. Some anxiety is normal, however, if anxiety lingers and starts to affect your productivity at work or in your daily tasks, you might have a more serious case of anxiety that would necessitate seeing a health professional.

Chapter 3: Emotional Stress

Let's look at some of the emotional signs of stress and what you can do to reduce and manage them.

Depression:

The Anxiety and Depression Association of America (ADAA) characterizes sorrow as a sickness in which an individual encounters a determined and extreme low mindset.

Research proposes a connection between significant levels of pressure and the beginning of misery.

One study of more than 800 ladies researched the connection between various sorts of pressure and significant misery.

During the examination, the analysts found that both constant and intense pressure occasions added to a more prominent frequency of sorrow in ladies.

Another observational study inspected feelings of anxiety of the working age populace. The members' general feelings of anxiety and side effects were estimated. Wretchedness was progressively basic in individuals who detailed more elevated levels of pressure.

Treatment:

• Reach out to a mental health professional.

• Both psychotherapy and medication can be effective treatments.

• Support groups, mindful techniques, and exercise may also help.

Anxiety

Anxiety differs from depression. It's portrayed by sentiments of overpowering fear, as opposed to only sentiments of pity.

In any case, similar to discouragement, thinks about have recommended that pressure might be connected to tension and uneasiness issue.

In one examination, analysts explored the impacts of feelings of anxiety at home and work on tension and melancholy levels. They found that individuals who experienced significant levels of work pressure were bound to have more side effects of tension and wretchedness.

Treatment:

- Reach out to a mental health professional.

- Treatment options include psychotherapy and medication.

- Alternative and complementary treatments are available for those who prefer a natural approach.

Irritability

Crabbiness and outrage can become normal attributes in individuals who are pushed.

In one examination, more elevated levels of outrage were related with both mental pressure and the probability of a pressure related respiratory failure.

Another study explored the connection between outrage, despondency, and feelings of anxiety in overseers. The specialists found a relationship between care-related ceaseless pressure and outrage levels.

Treatment:

● A variety of strategies can help keep anger levels under control. Relaxation techniques, problem solving, and communication are all great methods for helping to curb anger.

● Anger management techniques can help to reduce the stress in situations that'd normally leave you frustrated, tense, or angry.

Low sex drive

In certain individuals, a lot of pressure can negatively affect sex drive and the craving to be private.

A study distributed in 2014 found that constant feelings of anxiety negatively affected sexual excitement. The examination recommended that both elevated levels of cortisol and a higher possibility of being occupied prompted lower levels of excitement.

A great part of the examination encompassing pressure and low drive includes ladies, however it can surely influence men as well. One creature study indicated that social worry during adolescence influenced the sexual hunger of male hamsters during adulthood.

Treatment:

• Reducing stress can help to restore your sex drive and improve libido.

• Self-care, relaxation techniques, and exercise are a few ways to raise self-confidence.

• Improving communication with a sexual partner may improve intimacy and restore positive feelings towards sex.

Memory and concentration problems

In the event that you wind up experiencing difficulty with fixation and memory, stress might be a piece of the issue.

A creature study found that youthful rodents presented to intense stress experienced more memory execution issues than their non-focused on partners.

Another survey researched the pressure reaction pathways in the cerebrum and their impact on long haul memory. Specialists found that specific hormones following a distressing or horrible mishap can be able to disable memory.

Treatment:

• Various lifestyle changes may help improve memory.

• Maintaining a healthy diet and keeping your body and mind active can keep you focused.

• Avoiding activities like drinking and smoking can help keep your brain healthy.

Compulsive behavior

There has for some time been a connection among stress and addictive practices.

One paper developed that pressure related changes in the mind may assume a job in the advancement of dependence. As per the scientists, interminable pressure can change the physical idea of the cerebrum to advance propensity and enslavement framing practices.

Another concentrate even found that in specific individuals, hereditary varieties can assume a further job in the pressure reaction and weakness towards habit.

Treatment:

● Healthy lifestyle habits can help to reduce problematic and compulsive behavior. For more serious compulsive behaviors, professional help may be necessary.

● The National Institute on Drug Abuse has resources for starting on the road to recovery. These include lifestyle recommendations to help manage stress.

Mood swings

The numerous enthusiastic impacts of pressure can leave you having an inclination that you're encountering emotional episodes.

One study from 2014 inspected the job of different sorts of pressure tests on physiology, state of mind, and insight. The examination indicated that both social and physical stressors can have a big impact on emotional well-being and mood.

With the numerous other enthusiastic indications of stress, it's anything but difficult to see exactly how enormous of an impact pressure can have on your general state of mind.

Treatment:

There are many ways to improve your mood, such as:

- reducing stress

- enjoying nature

- celebrating with friends

- mindfulness techniques

For more serious mood swings that don't seem to go away, reach out to a mental health professional for help.

Chapter 4: De-Cluttering To Reduce Stress

You just might not realize it, but you might be surrounded by things that wear you down and cause you stress. It could be found in your bedroom, your living room, your kitchen, your car, and even your workstation; and it's called clutter. Clutter can drain your energy, distract you, and create chaos in your life. Imagine having a long day at work and arriving home to a house that's cluttered with dirty dishes in the sink, unwashed clothes on the floor, and a whole lot of unnecessary things in your living room—do you think you could relax and de-stress in that kind of situation? What about when you're already under pressure because your boss is breathing down your neck and you're trying to find a file that seems to have magically disappeared in your messy desk? Do you think that your cluttered workspace could help you in that situation? Probably not. If you want to

26

reduce stress in your life, one thing that you could do is to purge the clutter in your environment— at home, in your workspace, and in your life..

De-Clutter Your Home

It might seem overwhelming to start cleaning the litter in your home, especially if you've been used to living with it for a long time. However, even though you don't know where or how to start de-cluttering, the most important thing is that you do it. If you have a lot of clutter in your living space, what I would advise you to do is take things one step at a time. You could tackle one area in your home first, like your bedroom, for one weekend, and then move to the living room the following week. Here are a few ideas to start cleaning your home:

Think Simple

When de-cluttering your home, you should have a mindset to keep everything simple. Anything that you think is in excess should go away. Throw away whatever's on the floor, on countertops, and shelves that you feel are useless or that you haven't used for a while. Keep the things that you think are essential for you. One thing that you could do is to challenge yourself to fill up one trash bag. Go around your home and look for things that you could place in the bag; this will help you identify the things that are cluttering your home.

Donate to Charity

Do you feel like it's wasteful to throw away the excess things in your home? Why don't you donate it to Good Will? Take three boxes and label them with "keep," "donate," and "trash." Place the essentials in the "keep" box, the things that are no longer useful in "trash," and things that you think that other people could make use in "donate."

Follow the Three-Month Rule

This rule doesn't only apply to break-ups. Chances are when you haven't worn your clothes or haven't used your things in three months, then it's about time that you let it go.

De-clutter Your Workspace

Besides cleaning your home, the other thing that you could do in order to reduce the stressors in your life is to de-clutter your workspace. A study by neuroscientists from Princeton University reported that a disorganized environment such as a messy desk or disorganized files on your desktop could negatively affect a person's attention and performance, which results in stress. Another study added that clutter in the environment hinders productivity, creativity, and problem solving skills, which is important in a workplace setting. So what's the solution? De-clutter!

Clear Your Desk

The first thing you can do is to clean and organize your desk. Set a time during the week to clear everything off your desk and even out of the drawers. Take everything out and throw away the items that are no longer necessary. Wipe your place clean; you'll be surprised how much dirt you've accumulated! And then, before placing your things back, decide on a scheme for how you will organize things. For example, keep the small office supplies like pens, paperclips, and staplers in one of your drawers and place important files in another drawer; and then label them. The goal is to keep your desk clear; leave only your computer, phone, your planner, and maybe a framed photo on top of your desk.

Organize Your Computer

You might not realize it, but the cluttered files in your computer might just be adding to your stress at work. The files and icons that you keep on your desktop will not only slow your computer down, but also cause visual clutter. Organize your files in folders and keep the items on your desktop to a minimum. Delete any files that are old or unused. Remember to do this once in a while to keep your computer free of clutter.

De-clutter Your Life

De-cluttering your home and your workspace is a good way to reduce stress. Another thing that would help you to cope up with stress is to de-clutter your life. De-cluttering doesn't mean that you only get rid of the tangible things—you could also avoid situations that add more pressure to your life. Here are some ways that you could de-clutter and de-stress your life:

Learn to Say "No"

Even though you want to please everybody sometimes, committing to every opportunity might overwhelm and pressure you. Weigh your options and be wise in the things that you're going to commit to. You're only human and you don't have the power to do everything. So stop stressing yourself out; learn to say no.

Do Not Overdo Your To-Do List

Again, you can only do so much. Do not try to accomplish everything in one day. Doing this will only tire you out and cause stress. Keep your to-do list simple and learn how to prioritize. Keep the important and urgent tasks at the top of your list and the tasks that are important but could be done at another time at the bottom of your list. Experts advise that you write three to five important tasks in your to-do list; this will help you focus and accomplish things effectively.

De-Clutter Your Social Life

Like I said, de-cluttering also means that you get rid of the intangible "things" that are in your life, like being in a destructive relationship or being around pessimistic individuals. You might not realize it, but these things affect you and add stress to your life. Now, I'm not telling you to be a hermit. All I'm saying is that you keep only those relationships you have that are healthy and friends that motivate you and cause positive effects in your life.

How to Keep Clutter Out of Your Life

Even though you've successfully de-cluttered your home, your workspace, and your life, it doesn't mean that you're no longer susceptible to stress. The next thing you know, clutter, a.k.a. stressors, may be slowly creeping their way back into your life. So what's the best way to keep clutter out of your life? One thing that you can do is to create a system that will help keep clutter in check. Always evaluate your environment so that you can ask yourself whether or not you're heading again towards a cluttered life. You can schedule a weekly cleanup of your home or create a habit of clearing your desk before going home. The things I mentioned are only some ways that will help steer clutter away from your life, but the bottom line is that you should be on guard whenever you are starting to be overwhelmed with clutter again.

Chapter 5: How To Manage Stress At Work

Work-related stress can cause mental and physical damage to your body.

Learning how to manage stress at work is a good way to be a positive and happy person.

Workplace stress can manifest itself at your daily job but can be fueled by your activities outside of work.

Staying organized helps to keep knee-jerk reactions at bay when deadlines or feeling behind is an issue.

When you make it a priority to assess your stress level throughout the day, you can see big changes by taking measures that are preventative.

1-meditation releases stress:

Meditation is regularly suggested by medical professionals for stress relief.

Finding the kind of meditation that works for you is key in sticking with the daily practice.

If time is a concern yoga nidra is a meditation done in a sleeping position and teaches you to shut your body down, while you focus on your mind.

It is a guided relaxation that can help with a deep state of relaxation and letting go. Some practices teach that it is okay to do this to get to sleep, while others teach that it is imperative to stay coherent to focus on the mind and training it to relax.

This is just one example of deep relaxation through meditation, some find being in nature just as soothing as traditional meditation practices. Spend some time with yourself to find the right techniques that you can use to "let go."

2-get enough sleep:

Sleep is necessary for physical and mental health.

If you don't get enough sleep in a day, you may have a harder time dealing with stress and even lash out at people.

Making a schedule that allows for six to eight hours of sleep is important.

If you do not have the time because of other life events, scheduling long naps for the weekend may help you ease some of the weekly stress.

3-healthy minds love cardio:

Participating in an exercise everyday that gets your heart rate up will help you stay balanced mentally.

Many people choose to exercise in the morning before breakfast, so they can get the energy boost they need for work.

Ten to thirty minutes daily will help you release stress and be ready for the day. This can be running, dancing, walking stairs or whatever you like to do to get a short workout done. If the gym is something you like to do, join the many people who workout midday on their lunch break and get a boost during those sluggish hours after lunch.

4-become a morning person:

Your morning routine may be the culprit in how you handle stress throughout the day.

Make sure your mornings are not rushed and you are ten minutes early for work every day. This will allow you to enjoy the morning without having your whole day be about work.

Skip the extra shots of espresso and go for regular coffee, protein, and whole grains. A breakfast high in protein will help your energy levels during the day and whole grains help keep you full.

5-get it all out:

Find a buddy to vent to about your daily stresses at work.

Discuss your need to vent with a friend or coworker and set times away from your job to make a short phone call or text about the stresses you had.

Be receiving and helpful as they vent their issues as well.

Having someone to talk to about the problems you have and gaining active listening skills will help you resolve work stress faster.

6-take a break:

Once you have a plan in place to take care of yourself outside of work, it is time to concentrate on what you can change while you are at the workplace.

Many business professionals work through breaks or are salaried, so they don't get standard breaks allotted. Make it a point to take your breaks and mentally get away from your daily duties. Stretch, do chair yoga, walk around or eat a snack away from your desk.

Tech companies will provide workers with video games and ping-pong tables to take breaks from tedious projects, it is so popular that it is hard to find a technology company that doesn't provide fun ways to relieve stress for their employees. If there is a suggestion box at your company, this is a great way to help yourself and your coworkers.

7-soothing sounds with help you tune out stress:

One of the easiest ways to learn how to manage stress at work is to listen to music. The music should be relaxing and not disturb your coworkers. You may have to put headphones in or just set a small speaker on your desk at low volume. This will help keep you distracted and focused on being productive.

8-communication is key:

Communication is necessary if you are under severe stress with a project. Asking for help isn't always seen as bad, rather honesty can be a relief for your and your boss. If the key is to be productive and make the company money, you will do a much better job and probably faster if you communicate your needs and frustrations.

10-your to-do list might lead to procrastination and stress:

Your to-do list should be shorter. A long list of things can be daunting, which can cause some to shut down and/or stress about the things they aren't getting accomplished.

Try making three lists: a list that sits on your desk for today's objectives, a second list that needs to be completed by the end of the week, and a final list that needs to be considered in the future. The only list you see all of the time should be the list that needs to be completed by the end of the day. In the morning check your other lists and take an item or two to your daily to-dos. Keep your personal to-do list separate and hidden away at work, so you aren't distracted.

11-organization will make your day easier

Staying organized can make a drastic impact on combating workplace stress. Your work area should be clean and well stocked at all times. At the end of the day take a few minutes to empty trash, clean up your area and stock pens and paper for the next day. Keep a paper and pencil at your desk at all times for notes throughout the day, so you don't have to spend time trying to remember what someone said, or what you need to accomplish next. Take the time you need to get your emails checked at the end of the day and answer any questions others may have asked. All of these organization techniques will make the start of a new day easier and help keep stressors under control.

12-solitude:

When all else fails, get lost. Find a quiet place to work away from all of the stress. Move into the break room or request time in an empty office, so you can focus on your tasks easier.

If you are a manager or boss, let everyone know you will be back in an hour or two and work on a different floor in the building.

If you are not management, try requesting some time to work at home or a coffee shop a few days a week. Telecommuting is a great solution to workplace stress if your company allows flex time it is a good investment for your mental health and they save money on desk/office space.

Learning how to manage stress at work is easiest if one new habit a week is introduced. This will allow you to decide if it works well or you need to try something different.

Chapter 6: Lifestyle Habits Which Cause

Stress

Unhealthy lifestyle habits are some of the biggest stressors. You may not realize it, but some of the habits which you do on a regular basis could actually be a huge contributor to your stress levels. Do you lift a cigarette to your mouth whenever you're feeling stressed and anxious? Or, do you turn to alcohol to help you relax? Maybe you drink more cups of coffee in a day than you should, or stay up late working to find solutions to fix whatever is causing your stress? The thing is, doing any of these can usually only serve to make your stress worse.

Smoking

Stress and smoking tend to have a direct relationship with one another. For many people, having a cigarette is what they turn to when stressed as they feel that inhaling the smoke from the cigarette calms them and helps to clear their head. For smokers, being addicted to nicotine itself can actually cause stress levels to rise. When the body is deprived of nicotine, stress can be a huge symptom of cravings. Since having a cigarette quenches the nicotine cravings, the smoker begins to associate having a cigarette with feeling less stressed.

On the other hand, smoking marijuana can actually have the opposite effect. If you live in a state where marijuana is legal for either medical or recreational use, you may be able to try using cannabis to help with stress and anxiety.

Drinking Alcohol

The problem with turning to alcohol when you are stressed out is that alcohol is a depressant. Have you ever noticed that you are a happy drink when you were feeling good before you started drinking, but if you drink when you're feeling down, you only end up feeling worse? This is because alcohol tends to heighten whichever mood you were in when you were sober. If you drink alcohol when you're stressed, you could end up feeling worse. Along with that, alcohol can impair your judgement of situations, therefore getting drunk when you're stressed out could lead to some regrettable decisions. For this reason, it's vital to consume alcohol in moderation in order to help control your stress levels. For example, one glass of red wine per night can actually be good for your health, but it's important to avoid overconsuming.

Caffeine

In moderate amounts, caffeine can actually be good for us. It speeds up the metabolism and gives your body an energy boost, which can be useful in many situations. However, relying on caffeine can actually make you feel less energized, tired, and sluggish which in turn can lead to increased levels of stress. If you rely on multiple cups of coffee throughout the day in order to feel awake or have even turned to energy drinks or caffeine tablets, this could actually be causing you to feel more stressed. When your body's relying on caffeine for energy, you will experience caffeine withdrawal symptoms when you've not had your cup of coffee, for example – which can include feeling increased levels of stress. If you're relying on caffeine for your energy, it's important to cut down gradually. Cutting out caffeine altogether could lead to mild to severe withdrawal symptoms, depending on the level of your dependence. These could include headaches, aches and pains, feeling lethargic, and stress.

Sleeping Habits

Your sleeping habits are integral to your mental health. How well you sleep at night has a direct correlation to your stress levels. If you're getting enough sleep and at the right times, you will wake up feeling more refreshed and with a clearer mind to take on the stresses of the day. But, busy life and other things can get in the way of us having a good night's sleep. In order to make sure that you are fully rested and reap as many health benefits as possible, you should be aiming to have around six hours' sleep per night. Waking up early can also have some great health benefits, which is why you should look to sleep before midnight at the very latest.

Clearing your mind before you sleep is a vital part of making sure that you get a good night's rest. One of the biggest mistakes made by people in the modern day is to take their technology, which comprises a massive part of their lives, to bed with them. If you sit on your laptop in bed doing work or go through your appointments on your smartphone whilst you're lay in bed, your mind will start to associate getting in bed with working, rather than resting, which can affect your ability to fall into a restful sleep. Not allowing yourself time to relax and wind down when getting in bed can lead to issues such as insomnia or feeling tired and unrefreshed every morning. In order to get the best sleep every night, you should make your bedroom a tech-free zone after a certain time of the evening. Listening to soft music and using an essential oils diffuser can be great for setting the sleepy mood and allowing yourself to relax and float away into a deep and peaceful sleep each night.

Social Habits

You may not think about it, but your social habits can also contribute to your stress levels. The people who you spend time with and confide in can either be helpful or harmful when it comes to mental health, anxiety and stressed. When you are feeling stressed out, it's important to surround yourself with people who you can trust to give you the best support. Understanding how to ask for support and who to turn to can be hugely important when dealing with increased levels of stress and anxiety.

When it comes to being stressed out, it can often feel like some people know exactly which buttons to press in order to get your stress levels rising. Understanding who is contributing to your stress is vital to taking control of the situation and working on it. Sometimes, the people who cause our stress can mean little to us – for example other parents at your child's school, friends of friends, or people who work with you on the same level. On the other hand, sometimes it's harder to get away from the people who stress us out – perhaps they're your relative, or maybe your boss. In this case, it's vital to understand how they stress you out. Sometimes, talking to somebody who is causing you to feel stressed and explaining how you feel in a calm and sensitive manner can be helpful – not only will you feel better off for it, but it can also strengthen your relationship with the other person. Of course, it's important to remember that if you are going to speak to somebody in order to tell them how they contribute to your stress, you should do it in a tactful, non-accusatory manner so as not to further damage the relationship.

Chapter 7: Physical And Emotional Effects Of The Stress Emotional And Mental Effects Of Stress

Emotional Stress

Emotional stress is in its effects on the athlete that the more important the function. Emotional stress is that the stress brought to bear on the present psychological balance or psychological equilibrium of any individual; the indicators of mental stress will commonly be shown when the requirements of a situation are viewed as surpassing the private resources which the individual may bring to bear on them in an instant. Emotional stress differs from the Vast Array of psychological Health conditions, which are described, such as post-traumatic stress disorder or depression. Stress is a concentrated and transient circumstance connected to recognizable and well-defined aspects that are near the subject. Stress is a psychological illness. Stress is linked to the impending occasion that is current. Emotional stress Is Often considered a drawback Circumstance in living in addition to the game. It is the reaction of the individual to worry that decides the stress should be characterized. Many athletes mainly train to station their stress to positive effects on the results of an athletic event; this idea is better called "healthy strain." Stress is a composite of learned and automatic responses. Emotional stress represents a delicate balancing act to the athlete; even he or she's overly relaxed and not activated to reach the very best outcome if the athlete feels a significant position for little if any stress. It is improbable that a result is going to be gained after the athlete believes the effect of stress in a manner he or she can't restrain or exploit for advantage.

Stress arises in many conditions that are different for Athletic expertise opponents or Athletes, regardless of skill level, tend to feel the effects of stress profoundly. Stressful situations frequently result from numerous ailments, such as competitive stress, the desire, and the drive to succeed; coaching stress, the continuing stress of adherence to daily goals, mileages, or operation criteria; the outside forces made by teammates or coaches to attain; financial forces generated through the price of involvement in a game or as a livelihood component; or even the results of an accident, accompanied from the constraints of rehab or fears of recurrence. As a companion to the emotions. This illness, stress, has numerous physiological reactions. The majority of these effects are actuated by the human body's recognition of a harmful circumstance, which initiates what's often known as the "fight or flight" reaction. The brain signals the adrenal gland to release the hormone adrenaline as a reaction. Adrenaline makes an increase in blood stress and the pulse to some muscle activity that is essential. The body raises its blood glucose level, and blood flow is led into the body's extremities, preparatory. The release of adrenaline's results has been a decrease in motor management abilities and excitability. Assessing stress's consequences is of importance to achievement. Of importance to their capability and athletes to Separate, the positive facets of stress are that the distinction between instruction stress or bodily and stress. Physical distress and can be a supply of strain and exhaustion are inherent in the game. Physical fitness will work as a barrier to undue stress' consequences.

The channeling from the athlete of stress in that of a limiting requirement to stress can take lots of instructions; in understanding the principles underlying the management of stress in 43, a whole body of science has evolved to help the sports world. Sport psychology methods utilized to exploit the energy of strain center on the ability of the athlete to concentrate to the exclusion of all other distractions and thoughts on the occasion. Catchphrases like "blocking out stress," getting into the zone," and "positive self-talk" are resources utilized by athletes to place their heads in a perfect position to aid the entire body. Simulation is an important mechanism that is stress-defending, Helpful in athletic areas. Their stress on functionality will be reduced when athletes understand that the barriers to be confronted on a specific occasion. It's also imperative for an athlete to value the strengthening of a person's skills to offset the damaging consequences of psychological stress isn't an instantaneous process; stress-channeling approaches take the time to develop and need experience in their implementation, in precisely the same manner an athlete develops motor skills. Researchers in the field of psychoneuroimmunology (PNI) research the ways that the nervous system and the immune system communicate with each effect and other people's psychological and psychological wellness. Many studies are made to analyze the impact of nervous and immune systems. Though the area is relatively new. PNI research indicates that chronic stress can cause or aggravate mood disorders like depression and stress, bipolar illness, cognitive (thinking) problems, personality changes, and problem behaviors.

Stress And Depression

Byproducts of stress hormones can act as sedatives (compound Substances that make us calm or exhausted). When such hormone meds happen in massive quantities (that will take place under conditions of chronic stress) and they can promote a continual feeling of reduced energy or melancholy. Habitual patterns of thought that affect evaluation and increase the probability an individual will experience stress as negative (like reduced self-efficacy, or even a certainty that you're incapable of handling stress) may also increase the likelihood an individual will end up miserable. It's normal to experience a Selection of moods Low, in life. While a few "down in the dumps" feelings are a part of daily life, occasionally, individuals fall into unhappy feelings which persist and begin interfering with their ability to complete daily tasks, maintain a job, and also appreciate effective interpersonal relationships. The expression Major Depression is utilized to describe phases of depression that were unremitting, prolonged, and deep. Symptoms of big Depression might include: sleep issues; exhaustion; hunger changes; feelings of worthlessness, self-hate, and guilt; an inability to concentrate or make decisions; agitation, restlessness, and irritability; withdrawal from everyday satisfying actions; and feelings of despair and helplessness. Depression is associated with an increase in harmful activities and suicidal thinking and might make a person more vulnerable to developing psychological disorders. To learn more about depression, please visit our essential Depression topic center. Info regarding Suicide can be located within our Suicide Topic Center.

Stress And Emotional Disorder

Continuous stress can also impact Individuals with Bipolar Disorder. This illness, also called manic depression or bipolar affective disorder, entails dramatic changes in mood, energy level, and behavior in the highs of mania (one rod) into the lows of significant depression (the opposite rod). Mania is characterized by a euphoric (joyous, lively) Mood, hyper-activity, a feeling that anything can be possible, and an inflated sense of self-esteem. When in a depressive condition, people with bipolar disorder often experience a diminished need for sleep, racing thoughts, rapid speech (whereas the words will not come out quickly enough to keep up with their rushing ideas) and increased distractibility. Manic individuals, therefore, are more prone to engaging in dangerous or risky behaviors and actions and show poor judgment and impulsivity. People with Bipolar Illness change from ("cycle" is the expression used by mental health professionals)

Mania into the symptoms of the significant Depression, which we explained previously. People that are in a state that is miserable eliminate interest in things that used to give joy, create sleep difficulties to them, have unwanted stressed and sad moods, and always feel tired and exhausted, irritability, and or agitation, a short temper. Anger, guilt, failure, and despairing feelings could be experienced. Individuals with Bipolar Disease cycle involving and Mood conditions within the course. Functioning is disrupted by this mood biking, impacting judgment, action levels, energy, and behavior. Stress can activate a manic or depressive mood condition in somebody with a genetic vulnerability. A Bipolar mood event cans worsen when it's started; raising it is the strength and extending its length. To learn more about Bipolar Disorder, please visit our subject center.

Tension And Stress Diseases

May reveal mild Outward signs of stress, like biting, biting their fingernails, tapping their toes, etc.. In different peoples, chronic stimulation of stress hormones may promote intense feelings of stress (e.g., racing pulse, nausea, sweaty palms, etc.), feelings of bitterness and a sense of impending doom. Thought patterns that result in stress (and melancholy, as explained above) might also leave individuals vulnerable to extreme stress feelings. Dread or Stress feelings which persist for some time; that induce people to worry about forthcoming Scenarios (or possible scenarios); that contribute to avoidance; and trigger individuals To have trouble coping with symptoms of a single or Stress Disorders. Stress Disorders (like Generalized Stress Illness, Post-traumatic Stress Disorder, or Panic Disorder) are among the very Today, commonly diagnosed disorders. You can read more by visiting our Stress Diseases Disorders Topic Center. Specialized Info on Post-Traumatic Stress Disorder appears here.

Stress And Cognitive Functioning

The presence of stress hormones within the body may Change construction and the functioning of several facets of their system. More specifically, stress hormones can reduce the operation of neurons (brain cells) at a region of the brain called the hippocampus (a part of the brain that's essential for putting down new long term memories) and in the frontal lobes (the component of the brain that's essential for paying attention, filtering out irrelevant data, and using judgment to fix problems). Consequently, those that are worried may encounter and issues with decision-making, confusion trouble to find out new info.

Stress And Personality Changes

The term character is used to describe the constant Patterns of emotion, ideas, and behavior that characterize each individual across situations and time. Every person's character is regarded as influenced by either an inherited "hereditary" element (usually referred to as character) and from their interactions with the surroundings.

Some people today experience personality changes in reaction to stress hormones, which are a part of the environment.

The next changes in character aren't rare to observe in worried people:

Irritability

Hostility

Frustration

Anger

Aggressive feelings and behavior

Reduced interest in the look

The diminished issue with punctuality

Obsessive/compulsive behavior (attempting to deal with unwanted repeated thoughts or obsessions, by participating in compulsive behavior rituals like counting, checking, washing, etc..

Reduced work productivity or efficiency

Lying or creating excuses to cover up bad work

Excessive defensiveness or suspiciousness

Issues in communicating

Social withdrawal and isolation

Impulsivity (expressed as impulse purchasing, gaming, sexual behavior, or comparable)

The Physical Effects Of Stress

Everyone experiences stress. It's a part of existence, plus a small bit of fear may have some advantages.1, but too much stress may result in an array of unwanted impacts on the human body and head. Along with the effect of stress, research has shown it may exacerbate chronic conditions and impair resistance. Stress is connected with flare-ups of eczema, asthma, acid reflux, and headaches, and will to cause recovery times and frequent infections. Patient instruction on stress management could be underused though these connections are recognized.

More Colds

As a Healthcare provider in the health setting, Experience condition exacerbations and respiratory disease visits. I find the patients don't know why and come in with ailments or remember they've been getting sick. Sooner or later, I ask if they had some life events or individuals about work habits, and their lifetime, sleep. Frequently, patients will disclose they've been under stress. By way of instance, they are missing a loved one who could have experienced a separation or had any other stressor. Or, if it's not a strain that is psychological, it's physical. They'll acknowledge to working the graveyard shift or two tasks, running marathons, not sleeping, or suffering from physical stressors. As this relates to these cold or badly healing wounds, I consider this confession as a chance to discuss stress control. Research indicates that psychological stress may raise the risk of colds and respiratory ailments.2 Results from 1 study found that when individuals are under intense stress for"1 month but less than six weeks, [it] doubles an individual's risk of a chilly"3 and that "when individuals are under this kind of stress for over two decades, their risk of having a chilly quadruples."

Asthma Attacks And Eczema Flare-Ups

Eczema and asthma may have causes, but stress is one, which may be overlooked. Given the time constraints of appointments, suppliers could be fast slow to research and educate and to prescribe. Even though it does not have to be difficult for some patients to identify allergens such as cats, and causes smoke, stress is insidious. Patients might not be conscious of their state of becoming. Results from a study of children with asthma found that "the encounter of an acute adverse life event (e.g., the death of a close relative) increased the chance of a subsequent asthma strike by almost 2-fold. Children exposed to elevated levels of chronic and acute stress demonstrated a 3-fold gain in the danger of an assault at

the two weeks, which followed the event."
It's essential to take a moment Triggers, as
well as also the advantages of sourcing to
track the status. This might help discover
stressors and potential issues, thus
lowering the danger of. It is I have found
that patients might benefit from cognitive
behavioral therapy and may be under
severe stress or counseling. This approach
might help treat ailments that are physical
in addition to help enhance a patient.

Acid Reflux And Irritable Bowel Syndrome

It may perform as eczema, and asthma can
aggravate the same for ailments. Together
with patients' Criticism of nausea,
constipation, or gastroesophageal reflux
disease (GERD) symptoms, it's crucial to
talk about lifestyle. Including exercise
Sleeping counseling or drugs, stress
reduction methods, and habits To
decrease the degree of stress or stress.5
For individuals, Levels of stress may mean
taking more extreme steps such as
Changing tasks and professions or
identifying inherent mental health Like

posttraumatic stress, generalized stress disorder, or depression disorder (PTSD). The outcomes of a study Of Gastroenterology found in the people surveyed Had higher levels of stress disorders, depression, and PTSD.6 Therapy of These mental health disorders is essential in the treatment of symptoms.

Chapter 8: Visualization: An Excellent Stress Management Technique

You are suffering from a major case of stress, and you need something that will give you relief and visualization practice is just the tool you are looking for. Most of us have already heard or even practiced visualization before. Visualization is the act of imagining yourself in a safe and peaceful environment – a place that makes you relaxed, calm and happy. Different individuals find different things and events relaxing, and it is best to develop your own image of relaxation. There are mainly three important aspects of practicing visualization:

Practice: Remember, visualization is not normal, so it will not be relaxing to you straightaway. Generally, when practicing for the first time, beginners try to think of what they supposed to do and how they supposed to feel. This sort of preemptive thinking makes it harder for visualization to take effect. Practice daily, so this exercise becomes your second nature.

Involve all the senses: Involve all your five senses to the practice. For example, what does the place smell like? What does the place sound like? Preferably, you should feel the sensations, hear the sounds, see the colors, smell the smells and taste the tastes present.

Actions: Every visualization experts know that, occasionally, they will experience stressful thoughts. You have to find a way to change these distressful thoughts into something that you can get rid of.

For visualization practice, you can imagine a clear stream, a cool forest, a willow tree, a log cabin, a field of wildflowers, valleys, clouds, a sloping hill or just about any other scene that would relax you. Here is a guideline that will help you choose your relaxing imagery:

What colors exist in your scene?

Who is there?

What sounds are present in your scene?

How are you feeling?

What is the temperature at the scene?

What movement is occurring?

The practice

For the practice, I have chosen a sunny beach. Sit comfortably and relax. Close your eyes and take deep breaths.

You are driving towards the beach with the radio off, and car window rolled down. The sun in beating down on your lap and the wind is roughing up your hair. From your car, you can see people walking with blankets, and beach chairs. Most of them are wearing bathing suits and carrying drinks in coolers and food in picnic baskets.

You park your car and start walking towards the beach. You can hear the surf rolling onto the shore and smell the salty air. You avoid the crowd and go towards a quiet spot on the beach and spread your blanket. You feel tired after hours of driving and now pleased that you can allow your muscles to relax as you apply sun cream while sitting on the blanket.

You lie on the blanket with your feet extending beyond onto the warm sand. You are gradually becoming relaxed and continue to taste the salty air. You can now clearly hear the pounding of the surf and hear it ever so gently rolling back into the sea. Everything seems light and yellow and tan and blue. The sun's bright yellow, the ocean's vivid blue and relaxing ten of the people complement each other and seems just the right combination of serenity. You now have seen enough, so you decide to close your eyes and begin to take in all the sensations through your other senses.

Slowly the sun seems to move over your relaxing body. At first, your arms warm up as you feel the heat of the sun pass through them. You feel relaxed under the warm sun. Gradually the sun's rays touch your legs. The rays shift toward your upper body and now touching your chest as your entire upper body is now healed and relaxed.

The sun doesn't stop there. It rays shift toward your abdomen and brings warmth to the spot with it. The sun now moves toward your forehead, bringing warmth and relaxation there. Now your whole body feels warm and relaxed. Your body muscles are so relaxed that it feels like your body is sinking into the warm sand. Your body tingles from the sun's warmth, and you now feel warm and heavy.

You hear the seagulls as you continue to relax under the hot sun. They are free and light and peacefully flying over the sea. They glide towards the open sea and carry all your worries, troubles and problems with them. You are just thinking of your body's warmth, tingling sensation, and heaviness. You are now completely relaxed.

You have spent an entire day relaxing under the hot sun, and the sun is setting now. The sun slowly drops in the sea; you gently open your eyes, feeling brilliantly relaxed and content. You have no worries, no problems, and no cares. You open your eyes and look at the seagulls. They have taken all your problems and worries out at sea, so you feel gratitude, and thank them.

You feel alerted. Slowly you stand straight and stretch, the warm feeling is still all over your body. You feel warm, but rapidly cooking sand under your feet. You feel like a million dollars, and you think that the car ride home will be pleasant.

You are now contemplating your relaxed day while sitting in the car. You welcome this memorable, relaxing time. You say goodbye to the relaxing beach knowing that you can return to it anytime you want.

Problems with relaxation practice

Sometimes people face a few common problems when practicing deep breathing techniques.

Concentrating: Many People find it hard to concentrate while practicing relaxing technique. If your mind wanders off during the practice, don't get angry at yourself and gently turn your attention to relaxation process, just like turning a car.

Isolating muscles: Some people find it difficult to isolate muscles to tense. The cure is you have to practice daily. Just like any other skill, you need the practice to improve.

Worrying about time: Some people can't tolerate sitting and doing nothing (at least that what beginners feel). Again daily practice is the cure for this problem. If needed, use an alarm.

Chapter 9: How Does Stress Affect You?

The symptoms of stress can manifest themselves in many different forms, and they can be easily confused with other illnesses. There are physical, emotional, cognitive and behavioral symptoms that make themselves apparent after an overdose of stress hormones. These symptoms can range from minor to severe, but none of them should be taken lightly as they are messages to us that change is needed.

Physical

Physical symptoms of stress can be seen from minutes to days after a triggering event. These symptoms include palpitations, shaking of the hands, sweating, dry mouth, shortness of breath, tingling of fingers and around the mouth, frequent indigestion or heartburn, muscle tension and low energy. Some long-term side effects of too much stress might include upset stomach, diarrhea, constipation or nausea. Others might experience aches, pains, insomnia, frequent colds and infections, loss of sexual desire, ringing in the ears, cold hands and feet, difficulty swallowing and grinding of the teeth. All of these physical symptoms can lead to long-term illnesses.

Emotional

While most doctors and the general public can see the physical symptoms of chronic stress, there are emotional symptoms that can become debilitating. We may feel an irrational nervousness or unease that causes us to sleep less, lose the ability to relax and to become self-conscious. We may become easily agitated, moody, frustrated, overwhelmed, lonely or feel worthless. This can lead to an inability to relax our minds and, due to a loss of self-esteem, a desire to avoid other people. The emotional toll that stress takes on the human body will exacerbate the physical symptoms and should not be ignored.

Cognitive

Cognitive symptoms are those to do with

our thought processes and can lead to both emotional and physical symptoms of stress, as well as other illnesses. The cognitive symptoms of stress include constant worrying, forgetfulness, racing thoughts, disorganization, poor judgment, the inability to focus and being pessimistic. This can affect our life by causing us to become shut-in both physically and emotionally. While these symptoms may not be physically apparent, they are just as real and damaging.

Behavioral

When looking out for another person's well-being, learning to recognize the behavioral changes that might happen is important. Children may exhibit these signs of stress when they are feeling overwhelmed in life, but even adults will display these changes. We may experience changes in appetite, such as not eating or eating too much. We may procrastinate and avoid responsibilities. For example, a child may not do their homework night after night and an adult may avoid going to work and call in sick more often than necessary. Teens and adults may abuse alcohol, drugs or cigarettes in order to relieve their physical symptoms, but this is not a long-term fix and will cause severe problems in the future. We may exhibit nervous behaviors such as nail biting, pacing and fidgeting. All of these behavior symptoms are easily recognized when we know what to look for.

Consequences of Long-term Stress

There are numerous consequences of experiencing stress long-term. These can range from minor to severe and permanent complications. Mentally, we may experience depression, anxiety and personality disorders that can continue even after the chronic stress has been treated. It is important to remember that chronic stress can cause permanent alterations within our physiology. Physically, these alterations can include cardiovascular diseases such as high blood pressure, heart disease, heart attacks, stroke and abnormal heart rhythms. Eating disorders can lead to anorexia or obesity. Women may experience menstrual problems such as erratic cycles and extreme pain. Both men and women may experience sexual dysfunction such as impotence, premature ejaculation and loss of desire. Skin problems may arise such as psoriasis, eczema, acne and permanent hair loss. Also, as discussed before, physical symptoms relating to the gastrointestinal system may develop into ulcerative colitis, irritable colon and gastritis.

All of these secondary illnesses can be prevented if we recognize and treat chronic   stress.

Chapter 10: Limiting Beliefs Are The

Biggest Culprit Of Stress

What are limiting beliefs?

Limiting beliefs are those which limit us in certain ways to do the things. Due to our limiting beliefs only if I start to think I am not good enough. I can't do that. It is not meant for me.

Limiting beliefs are often about ourselves and our self-identity. The beliefs may also be about other people and the world in general.

In any case, they set the boundaries for us.

First you need to identify your limiting beliefs. Many people will tell you that this is difficult. It isn't.

You just need to figure out where in your life you're limiting yourself needlessly:

Where do you want to do something but don't, for whatever reason?

Where do you want to not do something, but do, for whatever reason?

When you hit some kind of limit, there's often a belief which defines that limit.

Secondly, you need to tease out the entire limiting belief.

This is also easier than you might think and doesn't require a lot of introspection, or soul-searching.

Beliefs have the form: If X then Y which means Z

For example, "If I try, then I'll fail, which means I'm a failure"

So go back to the things you identified in the first part.

If you did do the thing you don't normally do, what would happen?

This gives you the 'if X then Y' part.

Next, ask yourself what it would mean if that happened.

That will give you the 'which means Z' part.

Finally, you need to 'challenge' the limiting belief, or have someone else do that for you.

Fortunately, there are some general patterns which help to create change in a limiting belief. Here are two of them:

(i) Counter-example

Limiting beliefs are built from examples. If you can offer valid examples which don't lead to the limiting belief, you can begin to open up their world.

You'll need a number of good counter-examples, because one exception 'proves the rule'. Several exceptions show the belief is really shaky and requires redefinition.

(ii) Exaggerate

Sometimes a really vivid counter-example can make all the difference, so feel free to exaggerate to make your case:

"All dogs are scary? Even Scooby Doo?"

If you can get someone to laugh about their problems, you're already most of the way to changing them.

NOTE: When you challenge another person's limiting belief, be as gentle as you can. We're talking about the underpinnings of their reality here.

To summarise:

Limiting beliefs can be easy to identify and define fully.

Once you have done that, you can often see what you need to do to break them down - the cracks will begin to show.

Then you can overturn them and redefine your limits in the process.

We all believe in our New Year's resolutions, and Vows to each other. It's the inability to keep them operative that lets us down.

The mass-culture pundits all pretend that merely introducing people to concepts will be sufficient to overcome psychological, or belief, limitations. The largely unschooled mass audience believes them, and wonder why their lives return to usual after one to three months.

Once I recognized that I was hurting my life with my own decisions, I started to look around into both paid, and unpaid, sources of that kind of help. The paid stuff was powerful, and gave me an optimism buzz that then wore off. The unpaid stuff was almost as good. Everyone's life is about the book they are reading at the moment. That's what happens because the next occasion for doubt, or anger, or jealousy, or fear, or brain dumps, are just around the corner. Then life returns to the before temp-buzz paths.

This sounds ludicrous, yet is bitter, and destroys lives. A life is just as destroyed when repeated disappointment in failed efforts to improve result in resignation, and all of its ugly scenarios.

That reality was the motivation for many brilliant people in India, China, Japan, to come up with a way for people to reliably, in a self-directed fashion, without shaving their heads, or going to live in some colony, dissolve the limiting, and destructive beliefs.

There was progress, and that resulted in the founding of a group, in 1930, whose sole goal is world peace, and prosperity, through individual happiness. Here's a description of the method, and some concepts that underlie it.

Average persons often have far more ability to produce great results than they know.

The things that stop most people from being great are emotional, rather than cognitive blockages. If you can get skilled therapy, great, then the blocks can be dealt with in a systematic, and reliable way, by combining the therapy with this information.

If you can't get skilled therapy for your emotional blocks, you can still progress. Just get help from a senior practitioner who has used the method outlined below.

Here's some cognitive help.

1. You are unique, and so is everyone else.

Keeping this in mind will protect you from cultural, ethnic prejudice.

2. You need more than just yourself, in order to live, and so does everyone else.

Keeping this in mind will protect you from spoiling your relationships, and environment.

3. There are things you know, and a whole lot you don't. That's true for everybody.

Keeping this in mind protects you from feeling inadequate.

4. Nothing happens, unless the conditions for it to happen are right.

This knowledge helps to understand origins.

5. What goes around, comes around.

This simple sentence keeps you from making false assumptions about what to do.

6. Lives change, yet LIFE goes on.

This very powerful bit of wisdom helps to reduce the pain of impermanence.

7. We Don't Have to Be Perfect in Whatever We Do

This might sound obvious, but, I was raised by strict, middle-class Indian parents who only had only one dream for me — that I should have a future better than their present. To make this dream become a reality, they had sky-high expectations from me in whatever endeavors I attempted. Be it art competitions, dance classes, martial arts training, or school exams; I had to ace them all. If I didn't, they would make it clear how disappointed they were in me and how I had failed them.

These expectations continued to haunt me in my adult life, leading me to believe that no matter what I attempt in life, I had to succeed.

Don't get me wrong. Being ambitious is not bad.

But, wanting to win at everything to the extent that you fill yourself with guilt and brutal self-retribution each time you fail is toxic not just to your mental health, but to your emotional and physical health as well.

Failure in a small project that won't even matter in the ultimate scheme of things can bring your confidence down and make you feel like you aren't good enough.

That just because you failed in one project, you are a failure.

The truth is — you are not.

Every individual has their own strengths and weaknesses, and in the limited time that you have on earth, the best you can do is play to your strengths.

The endeavours that don't bring tangible results — let them go. Work on the ones that you are good at and keep improving till there's no one better at it than you.

After all, no one wants to end up like the old proverb — "Jack of all trades, master of none."

8.Making Mistakes Doesn't Make Us A Bad Person

You are only human. You can stop blaming yourself for that time you fucked up. Yes, I know you ended up hurting yourself and other people, but that was not in your hands. You did the best you could in the situation you were in. You don't have to blame yourself for the collateral damage.

You are allowed to forgive yourself. Guilt and self-hate will do no one any good, the least of all you.

No one is right all the time. And no one has to hate themselves for mistakes they now have no power to change.

Breathe, move on, and let the past be where it is. It is no longer in your hands, but your present is. Don't fuck it up over that one mistake you committed when you didn't know any better.

9. Spending On Things or Experiences We Enjoy Doesn't Mean We Are Incapable of Saving Money

Growing up, my family was not very rich. Eating out and going on vacations were rare treats, and the children were always encouraged to save as much money as they can. As a result, we used our pencils and erasers to the last millimetre, wore our clothes till they were torn or worn out, and never asked for anything that wasn't absolutely necessary.

This belief remained ingrained in me even as an adult.

I went through college living on the bare minimum and not regretting it. But when I started working, there was this one time when a group of colleagues planned a weekend getaway to a nearby hill-station.

My knee-jerk reaction was to say, "No" without even knowing WHY I had refused.

I could easily afford the money and the time for the trip, but even then, why did I not go along with the plan?

In a moment, the truth hit me — it all came down to my conditioning. I was so used to saving up every penny I could, that allowing myself small pleasures felt like I was being irresponsible.

Un-learning this lesson was the most difficult, but, with time and repeated practice, I managed to outgrow it.

If you are in the same boat as me, then let me tell you that you don't have to feel guilty about spending on things and experiences that make you happy.

Yes, you are allowed to splurge on that stunning wedding dress you had your eyes on for months. You are entitled to go on that 14-day trip to Tuscany with your partner. Spending money on small indulgences is not wrong, as long as you spend responsibly.

Maintain a savings account. Learn about personal finance (or hire an expert). Keep an amount separate for emergencies. And you are free to spend the rest of the money in whichever pursuit of pleasure you want.

10. Having Fun Doesn't Mean We Are Irresponsible

We can take breaks. You can allot time and energy in doing things that satisfy your soul. Just because your parents worked so hard that they barely had time to relax, doesn't mean you deserve the same.

Burning yourself out and working till you drop down dead is not the only route to financial success.

Take out time for yourself. Breathe. Indulge in a hobby, anything that makes your chest feel light.

But when you do this, don't go overboard.

Plan out your day beforehand so that even after all your tasks are complete, you have time left to spend on self-care.

Maintain a journal and list your priorities for the day. Make sure you include time for yourself there.

Prioritise self-care. Buy that set of scented candles that you worry might make you look silly in front of the store cashier. Get a professional massage session. Lie down, put on that face pack, close your eyes, and relax.

You are allowed to take breaks. And no, it does not mean you are lying to yourself or not reaching your full potential.

You're being you. And sometimes, that's all you need to do.

Image for post

Photo by Giulia Bertelli on Unsplash

11. Wanting Sex Is Not Shameful

India is a country of 1.3 billion people and 0 sex education. All my life, the only lesson my mother gave me was that sex is evil, and I should refrain from it till I am married. That my virginity is precious and I should safeguard it and give it only to my husband and no one else. If I fail to do so, no man would ever want me, and I would have to die alone.

I was young. Without realising, I had internalised this belief.

Fast forward to when I had my first boyfriend in college, and he wanted to get intimate. My mind said no, but my body wanted it. I had to exercise a herculean level of self-control and turn him down.

But, even then, later at night alone in my bed, I was racked with feelings of shame and guilt. I had been on the verge of giving it all to him. How could I be so irresponsible to want something so evil? How could I betray my parents and my future husband this way?

It took years of rewiring my mentality to reconcile my thoughts with what my body wanted. And if you have been trained to think along the same lines as I was, this is for you: no matter what the world might have led you to believe, the desires of your body are not evil. Carnal desires are just a way of celebrating the madness and mess that you are as a person. Holding back is like telling the universe you don't want to experience the gifts it has so generously bestowed on you.

12. Intimacy Doesn't Have to Lead to Heartbreak

All of us might have had bad experiences in the past where we gave all our love, time, and effort to one person, only to have them deny it, leaving us in a pool of our own self-pity and wasted dreams.

Relationships fail, and most often, there is nothing you can do to save them.

What you can do is not let a failed relationship define love for you.

John was a liar and a cheater. That does not mean all men are liars and cheaters. Sally had another man all this while, and you never knew. That does not mean all women have back-up options ready and will run off whenever you no longer offer them a "fair deal".

If you want to experience soul-stirring love, you have to keep your heart open to finding it, embracing it. Building walls around yourself to protect your heart will only lead you to miss out on all the wonderful people in the world who might be there right at the next corner.

The world is full of awesome, loving people, and you are capable of attracting them to you. Don't close your heart because of one failed relationship. You are in control of your love life, and when you choose to love and be loved. Nothing and nobody can stop you.

13. Admitting That We're Sad, Tired, or Sick Doesn't Mean We're Weak

Another pitfall of growing up in a middle-class Indian family is watching your parents get tired, but keep a strong face "for the sake of the family". My father would go to work each day, no matter how exhausted he felt. My mother cooked three meals for a family of four every single day without fail, even on days she was feeling under the weather. Seeing my parents work so hard imprinted this lesson deep in my brain: work is of the utmost importance. Anyone who shies away from work is weak.

But in truth, it is not.

You are allowed to skip work when you are sick. You are permitted to cancel plans when you are tired. You are entitled to seek help when you are unwell.

Knowing your strengths is excellent. But accepting your weaknesses, embracing them, and adjusting your life around them is even more liberating.

The ideas presented here are distilled from many centuries of efforts by many brilliant people. They are known all over the world, in diffuse, scattered form. Just knowing, understanding, and agreeing with the concepts will not change much below the surface of the mind-heart.The use of this method will not do what you want to get done. It will make you better.

Chapter 11: Effects Of Stress

As already mentioned earlier, stress is any response where your body needs to adjust and react to any environmental change. Your body reacts to environmental changes with physical, emotional and mental responses. There are many things you can do or some events might happen around you that might put stress on your body. Minimal stress can encourage you to do your best, help you to complete a given task under pressure and can even keep you safe in times of danger. However, when stress becomes overwhelming, it can do harm to your relationships, mood and can lead to severe physical as well as mental problems.

The problem with this modern world is that it is full of demands, pressures, responsibilities, frustrations and deadlines that makes people stressed to the extent they won't realize if they are stressed or not. Your nervous system doesn't really know how to differentiate between life-or-death situations and daily stressors. When you are stressed about traffic jams, being late to work, an argument with a family member or friend, financial problems etc., then your body might still react as it would have reacted to a life threatening event. When you constantly experience the flight-or-fight stress in your every day's life, it might bring about serious health, physical, emotional, and mental problems.

Health

Some of the health effects of stress include eating disorders or eating more or less, sleep problems, drug or alcohol abuse, reduced productivity, obsessive behaviors like counting or washing, nervous behaviors like pacing or biting nails, a weak immune system, neglecting responsibility or procrastinating, social withdrawal, hair loss, not feeling relaxed, making excuses or lying and can promote disease like heart disease, stroke, high blood pressure, asthma, cancer etc.

Physical

Some of the physical effects of stress include migraines or headaches, constipation, dizziness or feeling nausea, diarrhea, eczema or increase in skin irritations, chest pain, an increase in minor illnesses, loss of sex drive, feeling sweaty or faint and feeling exhausted all the time.

Emotional

Some of the emotional effects of stress include negative thinking, anxiety, being constantly worried, feeling overwhelmed, isolation or loneliness, loss of sense of humor, feeling overworked, increased moodiness and anger or irritability.

Mental

Some of the mental effects of stress include constant worry, confusion, difficulty thinking, mental slowness, forgetfulness, negative attitude, memory problems, poor judgment, poorer concentration and difficulty making decisions.

These are some of the effects of stress on our body, mind and general health. However, you should go for a checkup because they might be symptoms of other medical issues. I have mentioned them in this chapter so that you know them and create appropriate stress management techniques.

Chapter 12: The Benefits Of Stress Management

Stress can be one of the most debilitating emotions we can have. This is not only mental stress but also in many circumstances can lead to physical health problems - both short term and more long term in nature.

The sad thing about stress is often not so much the stress itself, though this is very unpleasant for the person who is stressed, but rather the fear of other people's reactions if the person wishes to confide in a friend, family or work colleague - even stress management specialists.

Another sad fact about stress management, and being a stress and anger management professional myself I know this all too well, is the widespread opinion that stress management does not matter; that it is a 'fluffy' concept that is not needed, or is only for weak minded people. From many years of experience now, I can tell you wholeheartedly that this could not be further from the truth.

We all know the effects that stress can bring about and if you are reading this in search of a cure, or at least some relief, from personal stress or that of a loved one, the effects of stress need no further explanation.

What I will do in this chapter is to suggest the main reasons why from my personal professional experience, 'stress management' can be a helpful course of action.

STRESS MANAGEMENT CAN STOP THE STRESS GETTING WORSE - An old saying comes to mind here that 'a problem shared is a problem halved'. From experience one of the main factors why stress is stressful, is that it starts off as something quite minor.

This problem whatever it may be is often 'swept under the carpet' hoping that it will solve itself which is seldom the case. As such it is then left and turns into a much larger problem.

By addressing the stress head-on can immediately stop this stress getting any worse - before stress reduction can begin.

Which course of action to take and rates of improvement depend on many factors ranging in time, nature of stress and of course for each and every one of us as we are all different. However, a reputable professional will tailor their approach to best meet the needs of their client.

STRESS MANAGEMENT CAN GET TO THE ROOT CAUSE OF THE STRESS - This is often not as easy as it sounds. Quite often the cause the stress is not actually what the person thinks. Stress from the journey to work every morning for example may not actually be the root cause of our stress.

This could be caused by a colleague at work or even something in our home life, but we have tricked ourselves into believing that this is the root cause of the stress because it is the simplest solution.

Left to our own devices, the probability is that we would not even begin to solve this stress and probably leave it as an underlying problem.

Speaking to a stress management professional can actually allow us to get to the root cause of stress - helped by speaking to somebody with wide experience of these matters, but also somebody outside friends or family - something I will discuss shortly.

STRESS MANAGEMENT CAN PROVIDE COPING TECHNIQUES FOR THE FUTURE - Getting to the bottom of the stress is one part of stress management but the other and equally important part of the process is gaining techniques for managing future stress.

It is often the case that speaking to a stress management professional, while being a great help and initially relieving the present stress; is of little use if the person is going to get stressed again in the near future.

Stress management therefore provides a means of providing each and every person the skills to relieve stress that may arise in the future - with the skills being tailored for every person. Therefore this stress management is not only for the here-and-now but also can greatly improve future well-being.

ENABLES US TO TALK TO AN EXPERIENCED PROFESSIONAL WHO IS COMPLETELY NEUTRAL - It can be difficult discussing anything with family and close friends, especially stress.

We may fear that family members will simply tell us they love us and that it does not matter, friends may be very biased, especially if it a family member or another close friend who is causing the stress and we may not want to tell work colleagues for fear of being seen as weak or unreliable.

Also with the current employment market we may simply not want to run the risk of losing our job if talk of this stress goes around the workplace.

Speaking to a qualified stress management professional confidentially has a number of benefits here - (A) all information is kept in complete confidentiality so that we can be as open as we like and discuss everything, (B) most importantly, the professional while experienced, will also be completely neutral.

Therefore there should be no fear of saying anything that will upset another family member or the professional taking the side of one person over another. They will simply sit back listen and judge the situation on its individual merits and provide the best advice possible having the whole situation discussed with them.

These are the four main reasons why, in my professional opinion, I think that stress management is a positive action to take if suffering from stress. As I have stated above, not only can stress management help with the current stress, but it can also help to pinpoint and solve other underlying concerns.

Chapter 13: Start A Journal

No, not the journal where you kept track of all your activities from childhood. Although that one can come in handy as a reference point. Start a stress journal. It will help you to identify all the regular stressors in your life. It will also show you how you've been dealing with them. So, each time you feel stress, take out your journal and jot it down. Write down what, in your view, has caused the stress. In case you're not sure, make a guess. Then put down what you felt, both emotionally and physically. Thereafter, state what your response was. You can also add what you did to make yourself fell better. As you continue keeping a daily log, you'll soon see common themes and patterns beginning to develop. Now that you've know what triggers your stress, you can start doing something about it. What strategies can you put in place?

Stress Management Strategies

Avoid Unnecessary Stress

Of course, not all stress can be avoided. It's also unhealthy to avoid a situation that you need to address. However, you may be surprised, by the number of stressors in your life that you can actually eliminate.

First, learn how to say "no" and mean it. Know your limits and endure you stick to them. This is regardless of whether it's in your personal or professional life. You can't be addicted to shopping when you're swimming in debt. Your boss can't make you work hours past the official duty hours. Don't say there's extra pay and you'll handle the kids and supper when you get home. You're not a workhorse. Taking a load that's bigger than what you can handle is a surefire recipe for stress.

You should also avoid people who stress you out. If you have a thorn in your foot, you don't walk around with a limp. You pull out the thorn. If someone consistently causes stress in your life limit the amount of time you spend with that person or end the relationship entirely. But don't be in a rush. Before you take this leap, first ensure that there's nothing that you can do turn the relationship around, Control of your environment. How? Do the evening news make you anxious? Turn off the TV. Don't want to be stuck in rush hour traffic? Take the longer but less-traveled route-there always one. Do you find trips to the market to be an unpleasant chore? Do your grocery shopping online. Since you know what causes you stress, find a way around it.

Steer clear of hot-button topics. Some people get upset over politics or religion. If a topic incenses you, cross it off your conversation list. Sometimes you may find yourself repeatedly arguing about the same subject with the same group of people. Simply stop bringing it up. And you can always excuse yourself when someone brings it up as the topic of discussion.

Review your to-do list. Take a close look at your schedule. Cover everything from workplace responsibilities to daily home chores. You may have too much on your plate. Clearly distinguish between the "shoulds" and the "musts." The goal is to take you off overdrive. Put the tasks that are not really necessary to the bottom of the list. Of course, if you're irrelevant you should eliminate them entirely.

Adapt to Survive

Sometimes you can't change the stressor. You can't fire your boss. You can't push forward your deadlines. You can't tell Mother Nature not to bring rain down on you on the day of your wedding. There are things that are simply beyond your control. And since you can't change them, change yourself. Do what you need to do adapt. How?

First, reframe your problems. Look at issues affecting you from a positive perspective. Hate the morning traffic? Use it to tune in to your favorite morning radio talk show. Look at your situation from above. Pay off your mortgage knowing that in the end you'll have a home to call your own. Take those college classes knowing you'll come out of it with a degree. Keep to your drug dosage knowing that you'll get cured. Ask yourself how important the stressful situation will be in the long run.

Perfectionism will drain you. Adjust your standards. No, your wedding does not have to be on a warm and sunny Sunday afternoon. All your relatives don't have to be there. And not all guys have t wear matching suits. Demanding for perfection is setting yourself up for failure. Set standards that are reasonable for yourself and those around you. When things are simply "good enough", learn to be okay with it.

Think happy thoughts. When something is stressing you out and bringing you down, try to focus on the positive. Reflect on your life, the party coming up that weekend, the promotion you just got, the joys of your marriage, the laughter of your kids, and even your own positive gifts and qualities.

Make Time for Some Fun and Relaxation

Beyond having a take-charge approach and a positive attitude on your life, you can reduce your stress levels by nurturing yourself. Take a break. Make some time for fun and relaxation. That way, you'll be in a better place to handle life's stressors. There are plenty of healthy ways to relax and recharge

Take a walk. Go for a hike in the woods. Call up your college buddy. Update your journal with the musings of your life. Take a long bath. Buy and light some scented candles. Relax with a warm cup of tea or coffee. Play with your pet. Do some garden work. Curl up on the sofa with a good book. Take a walk on the beach. Listen to music. Go on vacation. Watch a comedy.

Don't get so caught up in your everyday hustles that you forget to take good care of your own needs. Nurturing yourself is not a luxury-it's a necessity.

Set aside some relaxation time. In fact, you should include rest and relaxation in your daily schedule. And be mean with that time. Don't allow any other obligations to encroach on it. It's your time to take a break from all responsibilities and recharge yourself for another go at life duties. We'll go in-depth into relaxation later on, for more information on easily and effectively introducing relaxation techniques to improve daily life.

Connect with others. Meet up with your crew. Spend quality time with positive people who can enhance your life. Having a strong support system buffers you from the negative effects of stress.

Every day, do something that you enjoy. Make time for some leisure activities and hobbies that bring you pleasure. Go bird watching, spare time for stargazing, making your painting, or even working on your bike. Remember to keep your sense of humor. This also means you get to laugh at yourself. A good laugh is good for the spirit. The simple act of laughing will help your body fight off stress in various ways

Develop a Healthy Lifestyle

Eat a healthy, balanced diet. What you eat affects how you act. When you are well-nourished, you are prepared to cope with stress better. Hence, you should be mindful of what goes into you. Start your day right with a nutritious and satisfying breakfast. Continue to keep your energy levels up, and your mind cleared, by taking balanced, nutritious meals throughout the day.

Reduce your intake of caffeine and sugar. The temporary "highs" that caffeine and sugar give you often ends with a crash in your mood and energy. Hence, by simply reducing the amount of sugar snacks, soft drinks, chocolate, and coffee in your diet, you'll end up feeling more relaxed, and even sleep better.

Strengthening your physical health can increase your resistance to stress. Hence, you should exercise regularly. Physical activity plays a key role in managing the effects of stress. Make time for half an hour of exercise, at least three times per week. Nothing works quite like aerobic exercises when it comes to releasing pent-up stress and tension.

Remember to get enough sleep. Grabbing enough hours of sleep will fuel your mind plus your body. When you feel tires you have higher chances of increasing your stress as it may cause you to have and make irrational thoughts and decisions.

Alter the Situation

You don't always have to agree with everything the world throws at you. Not everything "was meant to be". If you can change your stressful situation, by all means go ahead. If you can't avoid it, there's no harm in trying to alter it. Figure out what you can do to change things. If you can, find a way to prevent the problem from presenting itself in the future. This often involves you changing the way you operate and communicate in your daily life.

Express your feelings openly instead of bottling them up. This applies to ladies "wanting to appear strong" and gents saying "it's weak to open p about your feelings". If there's something or someone bothering you, you should communicate your concerns in an open way. You obviously have to do it in a respectful way too. Don't just go insulting, punching or slapping the office clerk who's taking too looking to serve you. If you don't voice your feelings, you will build resentment. In addition, the situation is likely to remain the same.

Be willing to make a compromise. If you ask a person to change their behavior, you should be willing to do the same. If both of you are willing to bend just a little, there's a good chance you'll find a middle ground. You should also be more assertive. Never take a backseat in your own life. Face your problems head on. Do your best to anticipate, prevent or solve them. Do you have an exam coming up and you need to study? When your chatty friends show up at your door, tell them up front that you only have five minutes to talk. Or tell them to pop by later. Either way, don't knead yourself all the time.

This also applies that you need to manage your time better. Poor time management is a leading cause of stress. When you've stretched yourself too thin and are running behind schedule, it's hard to stay calm and focused. All you need to do is simply plan ahead.

Chapter 14: Breathe

When you feel stressed, it is likely that your breathing will increase. You also tend to breathe in a swallow manner i.e. from the chest. A deep breathing exercise should allow you to take fuller and slower breaths that reflect your true relaxed state. When you take slow deep breaths, you are likely to counter stress by slowing the heart rate, breathing, and reducing blood pressure.

To enhance both the physical and mental wellbeing and to keep chronic stress monitored, practice this 3-minute exercise at any time. The breathing exercise can help you decrease feelings of anger, frustration, or tension.

-Sit upright and ensure you are comfortable

-Pay attention to your current state and existence, and block those intrusive thoughts that creep up.

119

-Close your eyes and focus on your breathing. Inhale through the nose then hold your breath to the count of 4

-Exhale through the mouth and try to make the exhalation last 2 times longer than inhalation i.e. to the count of 8.

-Repeat the breathing technique for 3-5 minutes. If you enjoy the alertness and relieved state of mind, increase the practice session to around 15-20 minutes daily.

-Exercise regularly to achieve relaxation in stressful situations

Once done with the breathing exercise, slowly progress into muscular relaxation exercise for complete relief.

Progressive Relaxation

In this case, you will need to practically tense and relax each of the large skeletal muscles in your body. You only achieve the progressive muscle relaxation after you realize the contrast between tension and relaxation. You do this by increasing sensitivity of muscle groups that are more likely to carry tension.

Look for a quiet and secluded place, and then sit or stretch comfortably on the mat or mattress. Tighten each muscle then contract for 20 seconds and then release slowly. As you relax a particular muscle, pay attention on how the tension is released and the sensation you experience from relaxation. Begin with the facial muscles and progress to the rest of the body.

Forehead

Wrinkle the forehead and then arch both the eyebrows. Hold for a few seconds and then relax.

Eyes

Close your eyes tightly for about 20-30 seconds then relax.

Nose

Wrinkle the nose and flare the nostrils. Hold for some time and then relax.

Tongue

For the tongue, push it strongly against the roof of the mouth then hold for about 10 seconds and relax.

Face

Make an ugly and twisted expression on your face as if scared or amused. Hold the expression for 10 seconds and then relax.

Jaws

Clench the jaws tightly, then hold for a few seconds and relax.

Neck

Pull the chin down to your chest in order to tense the neck. Hold and then relax.

Back

Arch the back for a moment, then hold and then relax.

Chest

Just breathe as deep as possible, hold for 5 seconds and relax.

Stomach

Tense the stomach muscles for 10 seconds then hold the pose and relax.

Buttocks and thighs

Tense your thighs and buttocks for 15 seconds. Hold and then relax.

Arms

For the arms, tense the biceps, hold for some time and relax.

Forearms and hands

Tense the arms as you clench the fists. Then hold and relax.

Calves

Press the feet down, and hold for 15 seconds. Hold and then relax.

Ankles and feet

Start to pull the toes up, hold and then relax.

Realize those places where you feel loose or tight without changing the feeling. For a minute, imagine that each deep breath is going to this body part. Repeat the process and now focus on your body, while you focus on the sensations you feel in each muscle group. This muscular relaxation exercise should take around 15 minutes. You should do it two times a day, preferably for 2 weeks in order to get long-term stress relief.

Meditate

Whenever you meditate, you clear any information overload that has build up in your body to cause stress. This is especially because it helps give you a sense of calm, balance, and peace that helps your emotional well-being and your overall health. Actually, the benefits of meditation don't just end with a session; they last for a long time and help you to have heightened self awareness, helps you to build skills that help you to manage stress, helps reduce negative emotions and helps you to gain a new perspective on how to deal with stressful situations. In other words, meditation can help you to become more resilient to stress. So how can you get these benefits? Well, try doing the meditation technique below:

Start by finding a quiet and relaxing atmosphere (it could be indoors or outdoors) i.e. away from any distractions.

Sit in a comfortable position (it could be lying, standing, sleeping, sitting etc) then close your eyes once you are comfortable.

Take a deep breath while your eyes are closed then relax and wiggle your fingers/toes, loosen your neck, and shoulder. Ensure to harmonize this with your breath and then relax. Breathe in slowly and then breathe out and as you do that, imagine your problems/worries/stress leaving your body with each breath.

Strive to avoid all distractions if you can and then clear your mind. To do this, let go of your stresses, commitments, responsibilities etc and become self-aware. Just be in the moment and benefit from it.

Imagine/picture yourself in a happy phase. It doesn't matter what it is; it could be your graduation, your first date etc. Just see yourself happy.

Close your eyes then continue breathing deeply and then imagine every part of your body slowing down; this includes your heartbeat and your blood flow.

Continue in this state for as long as possible. And if you notice any distractions, try to bring yourself back by staring at a single point (it could be a hole in the room or a tiny object on the wall or even a candle).

Massage

Massage has been proven to decrease the levels of stress hormone cortisol. It also increases white blood cells, which means improved immunity. This means that a massage activates the body from the inside to help respond and correct any physiological imbalance, which have been brought about by stress in our life. You also get to relax, improve blood

126

circulation, improve sleep, and have an easy time in dealing with pain.

Massage also boosts the functioning of the lungs, boosts your well-being and improves circulation of blood throughout the body. In case you cannot do a regular full-body massage, you can opt for an occasional facial, manicure, or pedicure. These massage practices can nurture and treat your trigger points to relieve stress and anxiety.

Try this 5-minute self-massage in order to calm and relieve stress

-Begin by kneading the muscles located at the back of the neck and shoulders.

-Make a loose fist and then drum up and down the sides and the back of the neck

-Now use the thumbs to start working out tiny circles around the base of the head or skull.

-Use your fingertips to massage the rest of the scalp slowly. Tap the fingers against the scalp and move them from front to back, and later over the sides.

-Start to massage the face. Make a series of little circles using the fingertips or the thumbs. Pay attention to the jaw muscles, forehead, and the temples.

-Massage the bridge of your nose using the middle fingers, and progress to work outward on the eyebrows of the temples.

-Now close the eyes and cup the hand loosely over the face. Inhale and exhale easily for a moment.

- To make the massage more productive, incorporate massage oils such as almond essential oil.

Chapter 15: Quick Tips To Manage Stress

The tips in this chapter can be used on the spot anytime you begin to see the signs! These are short-term tips, but are effective in curbing stress. You can tweak them to your comfort level to best suit you.

Blow into paper bag and breathe

It might sound simple, but trust me on this one. You can take a paper bag and start blowing into it, as you breathe. Use this method either pre-stress or during the stress.

How it helps you? It normalizes your breathing and allows you to focus on a single task. Gradually, your breathing would return to normal, and the feeling of you being safe would kick in. You can then feel better and properly tend to the problem at hand.

Move away from the situation

You can hit a pause or choose to move away from the situation when it starts to stress you. Take a quick walk, or excuse yourself for a washroom break, or fake a call that you need to take.

By doing so, you give yourself a breather, and time to evaluate the situation. Don't let it get to an overwhelming state! Try to tackle it during the time you gain.

Destressing activity

As soon as the stress kicks in close your eyes, take a deep breath, start counting your fingers, rub your palm gently, try to visualize your clothes from top to bottom, and try to recollect your thoughts as you open your eyes slowly. Try to also reaffirm yourself by saying, "It is going to be okay, breathe, just breathe."

This activity deviates your attention from the worry and calms you. By counting your fingers, rubbing your palms, and visualizing, you communicate a sense of safety to your body that is needed to reduce stress levels.

Do these simple tasks

You can follow any of these simple tasks to reduce your stress levels.

☐ Drink water

☐ Listen to your favourite song.

☐ Chew a gum to relax your jaw

☐ Smell your favourite scent. (Citrus scents are best in reducing stress levels.)

☐ Watch a fun video

☐ Burn your favourite candle

☐ Buy some flowers

Vent it out

It gets overwhelming when the stress cycle begins, and you start to overthink, overanalyze every possible detail. When you vent things out, you gain a new perspective about them, and the feeling of insecurity recedes. You also realize how vague your overthinking was, and that none of it is going to happen. So, pick out any of the mentioned methods to release the tension.

☐Try to talk to yourself and break down the situation at hand.

☐Talk to a trustworthy friend and seek their help.

☐Write it down as you feel it and let it out.

Take a bath/shower

If you can take a shower or a bath, then I urge you to do so. Your muscles grow tense when stressed, so taking a bath can help you relax and relieve the tension. Use your favorite soap, shower gel, body butter, light some candles, put on your favorite music, and appreciate how lucky you are at this moment. Try to relax and think about beautiful things, things you are grateful for.

Practice laughter therapy

The laughter therapy is easy and gives you the best results. When you laugh, your body instantly produces the feel-good hormones (endorphins), which help in relieving stress. When you are stressed and alone, force yourself to laugh as loudly as you can. If you need some inspiration, then try to laugh in a weird way or mimic someone's laugh. If you can't laugh loudly smiling also helps in producing endorphins.

Get things in order

Clutter, unorganized space, and changes can also lead to stress. When you notice there is clutter, a mess in the room, or changes that you don't like, get up and get things in the order. Fight feeling lazy or shy and do what you need to, to feel better.

Go offline

Social media these days is the most common reason for stress. Someone not replying to your texts, comparing your life to others, constantly being available, a 24x7 distraction, and the need to please people every second of your life is stressful. When stress kicks in, go offline from all the social media platforms, be quiet, and center yourself in calming your body. Avoid any interaction that you aren't comfortable with until you feel well.

Take the drastic step

If your stress is due to bullying, abuse, or harassment, then take a legal action or report it to the authorities. Don't fight it in the quiet and don't deal with it alone. Be brave to take the first and the last step towards your abusers. If you feel that you can't report them, try talking to a trustworthy source, a general practitioner, guidance counsellor, a support group. Reach out for help.

Sing a song

You might be surprised how singing can release tension and help you to feel more weightless! A good singer, a not-so-good singer, just sing! In the comfort of your room, while you talk a walk, or as you jam out to your iPod. Find a song you like, or make one up. Give this a go and you might notice your day become a little brighter.

Get a massage

A massage is the most calming thing that you can try to de-stress your body and soul. It makes you feel pampered and rested. It relaxes the knots and tensed muscles. Massages often help in releasing tied up emotions (stress) in the body. Try to schedule a massage once a week, if you are highly stressed, it makes a drastic difference.

Bask in the sun

Vitamin D helps the body in relieving stress. If you have a vitamin D deficiency, you will experience higher levels of stress. Sun is a source of vitamin D. Make it a habit to sit under the sun for 10 minutes during the day. Sitting in the sun also uplifts your mood and makes you feel better.

Reassure yourself

Always reassure yourself with the belief, that the things will get better. Keep your self- confidence, and faith high, as it will help you in dealing with tough times. Remember memories in the past during tough times of your life, and evaluate how you overcame those situations. Believe in yourself and don't give up.

Zoom out of life

We become stressed when we think too highly of ourselves, thinking that everything is under our control. Stress tends to build when we make the problem larger than life and continue overanalyzing it. You must try to look at the bigger picture of your life. Don't stress about small things! Most of those things we freak out about don't even matter that much. Control the things you can control. That way, you can see the bigger picture and it isn't so daunting.

Buy/adopt a pet

If you experience high levels of stress, buy or adopt a pet! Through providing unlimited cuddles, love, company, and support, many people have noticed a drastic drop in their stress levels after welcoming a pet into their life.

Surround yourself with nature

Nature heals the soul and refreshes the mind. If you are stressed, take a long walk or bike into the woods, mountain trails, or a scenic park, and experience nature. Appreciate the beauty you live under! You can also incorporate plants in your house or workspace, or hey, maybe you'd like to try gardening.

These are a few quick tips that are highly effective in dealing with stress, on the spot. Which of these fit best with your life? What is something new you could try?

Chapter 16: Alleviating Chronic Stress

Stress often creeps into our lives and finds a way into our body and mind. When that happens, our wellbeing is disrupted. Unfortunately, no matter how much you try to prevent it, some stress will still accumulate in your life.

While you can never completely get rid of stress, you can learn to tackle it in positive ways. To keep stress from building up in your life, you have to alleviate it.

Know Your Stressors

First and most important, find out what triggers your stress. For a few days, pay close attention to how you feel throughout the day and how different situations, activities, and people affect your emotions. This will help you become more aware of your stressors. For instance, if your stress is work related, find out the core reason behind that stress. Is it because you do not like your job or because you feel over-burdened?

After identifying your stressor, try to manage it as much as you can. If not meeting deadlines stresses you, try to focus more on your projects so you can accomplish work related tasks on time and in the process, alleviate stress.

To understand your stressors better so you can manage them effectively, be aware of what upsets you and stirs up negativity in you. In addition to avoiding your stressors and finding ways to fix them, try the following hacks to alleviate your stress too so you feel calm as soon as you sense stress accumulating inside you.

Relax Your Mind

Relaxing your mind helps you stay calm and composed. If you build a habit of resting your racing mind, you will begin to block stress. Here are a few strategies that can help you soothe your racing mind and give it a break from excessive thinking:

Meditation

Meditation is by far one of the best ways to induce mindfulness, which as stated before, is the best way to live in the present. Mindfulness helps you stay more aware of yourself and your thoughts, thus keeping you from falling into the trap of negative thoughts.

Meditation helps calm your racing mind thus bringing your focus to the present moment. As you let go of all your worries, you find yourself becoming peaceful. This happens mainly because meditation helps bring your brainwaves from an active state to a calmer one.

Your brain has five brainwave states, each with a different set of frequencies and different effects on your mind and body. These brainwave states are **gamma, beta, alpha, theta,** and **delta** with gamma being the most active and delta being the least active.

The gamma and beta states help you with planning and active decision-making but when over energized, these states can result in chronic stress, anxiety, and depression. Alpha, theta, and delta are the more peaceful brainwave states that help you relax.

Meditation calms your racing mind bringing it from the gamma or beta state to the alpha, delta, or even theta state. When your racing mind calms down, you gain clarity and a peace of mind that helps you think clearly.

To enjoy these benefits, make meditation part of your routine.

While there are many ways to meditate, one of the simplest ways is to practice 'mindfulness breathing meditation.' Here is how you can practice it.

Sit comfortably in a peaceful room and close your eyes.

Let your mind calm down by thinking of anything peaceful such as the feeling you have when you hug your partner.

As you feel better, bring your attention to your breath and focus on it and nothing else.

In your mind, say, "I am with my in-breath" as you inhale and as you exhale, "I am with my out-breath"

Keep doing this for 5 minutes or more and you will start feeling more peaceful than before.

When your thoughts divert to something else, gently tell yourself that you must focus on your breath right now and bring your attention back to your breath. Do this as many times as your mind wanders off in thought and soon (maybe not in the first few sessions), you will find it easy to focus on your breath.

Practice this exercise daily and with time, you will get better at it. When you find it easy to meditate for 5 minutes, increase the duration of your session. As you practice for longer periods, you will slowly develop the ability to become more aware of your thoughts and discern a debilitating thought from a constructive one. That is exactly the ability that helps you identify stress-triggering thoughts and manage them on time.

In addition to meditation, self-hypnosis is another practice that helps calm you down and eliminate stress.

Self-Hypnosis

Self-hypnosis is a state of mind that occurs naturally and many often describe it as a sharp state of concentration. With this practice, you can easily calm your mind and change your thinking pattern, which in turn helps you alleviate stress and become more peaceful. Here is how you can practice it.

Lie down comfortably and close both your eyes. Take a few deep breaths to calm yourself down.

When you feel calm, pick any point on the wall in front of you or any object to focus on.

Completely focus on your point of focus and let your eyes feel heavy.

As your eyelids feel heavy, chant a suggestion you want to imbed in your subconscious. If you want to feel peaceful and happy, say, "I am relaxed and happy." Choose any affirmation you want just as you do when practicing incantation.

Keep chanting that suggestion, focus on it in your mind, and keep looking at the point of focus in front of you until your eyes close.

Notice any sort of tension in your mind and get rid of it by imagining it going out of your body.

As you feel calmer, think that you are at the top of a staircase with 10 steps.

Imagine moving down the flight of stairs and as you move to the sixth step, you start submerging into water as the staircase is submerged into water from the sixth step until the first.

As you move down the stairs, focus on each step and repeat its number in your head.

Tell yourself that you are moving from a state of impurity and stress to one of complete bliss and serenity.

Enjoy the state of purity as you finally step on the first step. Make sure you completely involve yourself in the scenario by focusing on tiny details such as the color of the staircase and the different sensations you experience as you move down.

Relish the state of peace as you step on the first step and make sure you keep chanting your affirmation throughout the practice.

When you feel great, exit the hypnotic state; move from the first step to the 10th step.

Carry out all these steps a few times to imbed the positive affirmation into your subconscious so it relaxes your strained mind.

Practice this regularly until you master the art of self-hypnosis. Soon, you will find yourself experiencing complete relief from stress through this technique.

Deep Breathing

Shallow breathing is one of the biggest triggers of stress and anxiety. As your sympathetic nervous system activates, it produces different psychological changes in your body including rapid breathing that makes you feel stressed.

To alleviate stress, train yourself to breathe deeply. When you naturally breathe deeply, you do not allow yourself to fall in the trap of shallow breathing and subsequently, you stay calm.

Here is an easy deep breathing practice you can practice daily to build a habit of it.

Take a deep in-breath for a count of 7 and hold that breath for another count of 7. Breathe through your nose and completely fill in your abdomen with air.

When your abdomen becomes full with air, slowly and deeply exhale all that air to another count of 7.

Keep doing this for 2 to 5 minutes to let go of the strain building up in your mind and body.

Make sure you exercise this practice twice daily and then slowly do it more often so you train yourself to breathe deeply at all times.

Drink Lots of Water

Science shows that staying hydrated helps combat stress. Hydrating your body helps lower the cortisol levels in your body. When there is less cortisol in your bloodstream, your stress levels start to reduce too.

To assuage chronic stress, make a habit of drinking at least 2 to 3 liters of clean water. By drinking a tall glass of cool water as soon as you feel stressed, you will instantly feel relaxed.

If consuming too much plain water is tough for you, increase your intake of foods rich in water; such foods include watermelons, tomatoes, cabbage, and cucumbers.

Do Something Relaxing at the End of the Day

With the different responsibilities and tasks you have to execute during the day, you are bound to feel exhausted by evening. To get rid of that stress, make sure to do something pleasant and relaxing before your day ends. This helps you end your day on a happy note leaving you fresh and energized.

You could spend time with loved ones, go for a nice soothing walk, listen to your favorite music and dance, watch your all-time favorite movie, or do anything else that makes you feel happy. Ensure you do this daily to build a habit of ending your day on a good, happy note.

Build a stress-free zone and spend some quality time in that zone every day. Your stress-free zone could be your bedroom, a corner in your garden or any inviting space in your house that makes you feel peaceful and warm. Put your favorite things in that area and clear it of anything that stresses you.

Try Some Natural Remedies

Two of the best natural remedies you can use to curb stress are to take a warm bath with Epsom salt and to drink chamomile tea regularly. Epsom salt is rich in magnesium that increases the levels of serotonin in your body (mood improving neurotransmitter) and helps fight stress. Mix a cup of Epsom salt and a few drops of your favorite essential oil in a bathtub full of warm water. Lie in the bathtub and enjoy this soothing bath for 20 to 30 minutes. Do this regularly and especially before bed to feel calm and energized.

Chamomile has a sedating effect on your nervous system and relaxes you within minutes. Drink a cup of it an hour or two before going to bed to enjoy a good night's sleep.

Improve Your Posture

Research shows that poor posture, and regularly carrying yourself in low power poses increases the cortisol levels in your body and lowers testosterone levels. This occurs in both men and women. If you carry yourself in low power poses, you cross your arms and legs, you walk or sit hunched over or your shoulders sag. A low power pose is essentially your body taking up the least amount of space possible. Carrying yourself in low power poses affects your confidence and emotional wellbeing. Pay close attention to your posture and if you are in the habit of practicing low power poses, switch to high power poses.

For both men and women, high levels of testosterone increase confidence and low levels of cortisol lead to decreased anxiety along with the ability to alleviate stress. If you carry yourself in high power poses, your hands are on your hips or laced behind your head or your legs are stretched out. Strive to carry yourself in high power poses where your limbs spread out and take up more space.

High power or open postures convey power and low power or closed postures convey little power.

Become Active

An active lifestyle is a fabulous way to reduce and eliminate stress. Science shows that staying active increases the production of feel good neurotransmitters such as dopamine and serotonin in your body. These hormones lower your stress and help you feel relaxed. To enjoy the effects of these neurotransmitters, stay as active as you can.

Exercise for as little as 10 minutes daily. 10 minutes is not too long so squeezing in a 10-minute exercise or physical activity in your routine should not be that difficult. If hitting the gym or doing traditional exercises is tough for you, do any vigorous physical activity you enjoy such as walking, swimming, yoga, aerobics, or cycling.

Instead of taking the elevator, take the stairs. The more you move, the more in control you are of your stress levels.

When you make these practices daily habits, you will start to alleviate stress. However, to eliminate stress for good, incorporate the strategies discussed in the next chapter in your life.

Chapter 17: Relaxation Techniques

We have already talked about the unhealthy ways to relieve stress, so now its time to discuss the good ways to relieve stress. Relaxing is the best way to relieve stress, but you need to know how to do it in a healthy way. Below are some ways to relax and deal with stress in healthy or productive ways.

Talk to someone about what you are going through. Sometimes just talking to someone about your problem will make you feel better, even if they can't do anything to help the situation. Its helps to know that someone cares enough to listen.

Listen to soothing music. It can calm you and give you the time you need to think things through.

Try deep breathing exercises. It helps by relaxing you and getting more oxygen to your brain. It also lowers heart rate and blood pressure. Breathe slowly in through your nose and out through your mouth.

Do something creative. This can be anything you enjoy doing like playing an instrument, drawing, or painting. It will take your mind off of your problems and relax you so that you can think more clearly.

Exercise is one of the best things you can do to relax yourself and it also has great health benefits for you.

Meditate. Meditating for 5-10 minutes can help reduce stress. A repetitive mantra can also make it easier to focus while you are meditating.

Slow down. If you start feeling overwhelmed or stressed, just slow down. Live in the moment. Think only about what you are doing at that moment. If you are eating, enjoy the taste of your food. Focus on one thing.

Listen to rock or pop music. If you are angry or anxious, listening to loud music can be just what you needed. Feel free to sing and dance along.

Get a massage. A massage can relax not only your body but also your mind.

Hypnosis. Sometime other relaxation techniques don't work for everyone. If you need to think outside the box or are just interested to see how it works, try hypnosis.

Anything that you do that helps you relax and also benefits you is a healthy relaxation technique. Try different things until you find something that fits you. Make sure to use your relaxation techniques in addition to positive coping skills such as positive thinking, problem solving, and time management.

Chapter 18: Relaxation Techniques For

Stress Relief

To effectively combat stress, you need to activate your body's natural relaxation response. Techniques such as deep breathing, visualization, meditation, and yoga can help.

Finding The Best Relaxation Technique For You

For many of us, relaxation means flopping on the couch and zoning out in front of the TV at the end of a stressful day. But this does little to reduce the damaging effects of stress. Rather, you need to activate your body's natural relaxation response, a state of deep rest that puts the brakes on stress, slows your breathing and heart rate, lowers your blood pressure, and brings your body and mind back into balance. You can do this by practicing relaxation techniques such as deep breathing, meditation, rhythmic exercise, yoga, or tai chi.

While you may choose to pay for a professional massage or acupuncture session, for example, most relaxation techniques can be done on your own or with the aid of a free audio download or inexpensive smartphone app. It's important to remember, however, that there is no single relaxation technique that works for everyone. We're all different. The right technique is the one that resonates with you, fits your lifestyle, and is able to focus your mind to elicit the relaxation response. That means, it may require some trial and error to find the technique (or techniques) that work best for you. Once you do, regular practice can help reduce everyday stress and anxiety, improve your sleep, boost your energy and mood, and improve your overall health and wellbeing.

Relaxation Technique

Deep Breathing

With its focus on full, cleansing breaths, deep breathing is a simple yet powerful relaxation technique. It's easy to learn, can be practiced almost anywhere, and provides a quick way to get your stress levels in check. Deep breathing is the cornerstone of many other relaxation practices, too, and can be combined with other relaxing elements such as aromatherapy and music. While apps and audio downloads can guide you through the process, all you really need is a few minutes and a place to sit quietly or stretch out.

How to practice deep breathing

• Sit comfortably with your back straight. Put one hand on your chest and the other on your stomach.

• Breathe in through your nose. The hand on your stomach should rise. The hand on your chest should move very little.

• Exhale through your mouth, pushing out as much air as you can while contracting your abdominal muscles. The hand on your stomach should move in as you exhale, but your other hand should move very little.

• Continue to breathe in through your nose and out through your mouth. Try to inhale enough so that your lower abdomen rises and falls. Count slowly as you exhale.

If you find it difficult breathing from your abdomen while sitting up, try lying down. Put a small book on your stomach, and breathe so that the book rises as you inhale, and falls as you exhale.

Why breathe from your belly?

Belly breathing stimulates the vagus nerve, which runs from the head down the neck, through the chest, and to the colon. This activates your relaxation response, reducing your heart rate and blood pressure and lowering stress levels.

Progressive Muscle Relaxation

Progressive muscle relaxation is a two-step process in which you systematically tense and relax different muscle groups in the body. With regular practice, it gives you an intimate familiarity with what tension—as well as complete relaxation—feels like in different parts of your body. This can help you react to the first signs of the muscular tension that accompanies stress. And as your body relaxes, so will your mind.

Progressive muscle relaxation can be combined with deep breathing for additional stress relief.

Practicing Progressive Muscle Relaxation

Consult with your doctor first if you have a history of muscle spasms, back problems, or other serious injuries that may be aggravated by tensing muscles.

Start at your feet and work your way up to your face, trying to only tense those muscles intended.

• Loosen clothing, take off your shoes, and get comfortable.

• Take a few minutes to breathe in and out in slow, deep breaths.

160

• When you're ready, shift your attention to your right foot. Take a moment to focus on the way it feels.

• Slowly tense the muscles in your right foot, squeezing as tightly as you can. Hold for a count of 10.

• Relax your foot. Focus on the tension flowing away and how your foot feels as it becomes limp and loose.

• Stay in this relaxed state for a moment, breathing deeply and slowly.

• Shift your attention to your left foot. Follow the same sequence of muscle tension and release.

• Move slowly up through your body, contracting and relaxing the different muscle groups.

• It may take some practice at first, but try not to tense muscles other than those intended.

Progressive Muscle Relaxation Sequence

1. Right foot, then left foot

2. Right calf, then left calf

3. Right thigh, then left thigh

4. Hips and buttocks

5. Stomach

6. Chest

7. Back

8. Right arm and hand, then left arm and hand

9. Neck and shoulders

10. Face

Body Scan Meditation

This is a type of meditation that that focuses your attention on various parts of your body. Like progressive muscle relaxation, you start with your feet and work your way up. But instead of tensing and relaxing muscles, you simply focus on the way each part of your body feels, without labeling the sensations as either "good" or "bad."

• Lie on your back, legs uncrossed, arms relaxed at your sides, eyes open or closed. Focus on your breathing for about two minutes until you start to feel relaxed.

• Turn your focus to the toes of your right foot. Notice any sensations you feel while continuing to also focus on your breathing. Imagine each deep breath flowing to your toes. Remain focused on this area for three to five seconds (or more).

• Move your focus to the sole of your right foot. Tune in to any sensations you feel in that part of your body and imagine each breath flowing from the sole of your foot. After one or two minutes, move your focus to your right ankle and repeat. Move to your calf, knee, thigh, hip, and then repeat the sequence for your left leg. From there, move up the torso, through the lower back and abdomen, the upper back and chest, and the shoulders. Pay close attention to any area of the body that causes you pain or discomfort.

• After completing the body scan, relax for a while in silence and stillness, noting how your body feels. Then slowly open your eyes and stretch, if necessary.

Visualization

Visualization, or guided imagery, is a variation of traditional meditation that involves imagining a scene in which you feel at peace, free to let go of all tension and anxiety. Choose whatever setting is most calming to you, whether it's a tropical beach, a favorite childhood spot, or a quiet wooded glen.

You can practice visualization on your own or with an app or audio download to guide you through the imagery. You can also choose to do your visualization in silence or use listening aids, such as soothing music or a sound machine or a recording that matches your chosen setting: the sound of ocean waves if you've chosen a beach, for example.

Practicing Visualization

Close your eyes and imagine your restful place. Picture it as vividly as you can: everything you see, hear, smell, taste, and feel. Just "looking" at it in your mind's eye like you would a photograph is not enough. Visualization works best if you incorporate as many sensory details as possible. For example, if you are thinking about a dock on a quiet lake:

• See the sun setting over the water

• Hear the birds singing

• Smell the pine trees

• Feel the cool water on your bare feet

• Taste the fresh, clean air

Enjoy the feeling of your worries drifting away as you slowly explore your restful place. When you are ready, gently open your eyes and come back to the present. Don't worry if you sometimes zone out or lose track of where you are during a visualization session. This is normal. You may also experience feelings of heaviness in your limbs, muscle twitches, or yawning. Again, these are normal responses.

Self-Massage

You're probably already aware how much a professional massage at a spa or health club can help reduce stress, relieve pain, and ease muscle tension. What you may not be aware of is that you can experience some of the same benefits at home or work by practicing self-massage, or trading massages with a loved one.

Try taking a few minutes to massage yourself at your desk between tasks, on the couch at the end of a hectic day, or in bed to help you unwind before sleep. To enhance relaxation, you can use aromatic oil, scented lotion, or combine self-message with mindfulness or deep breathing techniques.

A Five-Minute Self-Massage To Relieve Stress

A combination of strokes works well to relieve muscle tension. Try gentle chops with the edge of your hands or tapping with your fingers or cupped palms. Put fingertip pressure on muscle knots. Knead across muscles, and try long, light, gliding strokes. You can apply these strokes to any part of the body that falls easily within your reach. For a short session like this, try focusing on your neck and head:

• Start by kneading the muscles at the back of your neck and shoulders. Make a loose fist and drum swiftly up and down the sides and back of your neck. Next, use your thumbs to work tiny circles around the base of your skull. Slowly massage the rest of your scalp with your fingertips. Then tap your fingers against your scalp, moving from the front to the back and then over the sides.

• Now massage your face. Make a series of tiny circles with your thumbs or fingertips. Pay particular attention to your temples, forehead, and jaw muscles. Use your middle fingers to massage the bridge of your nose and work outward over your eyebrows to your temples.

• Finally, close your eyes. Cup your hands loosely over your face and inhale and exhale easily for a short while.

Mindfulness Meditation

Mindfulness has become extremely popular in recent years, garnering headlines and endorsements from celebrities, business leaders, and psychologists alike. So, what is mindfulness? Rather than worrying about the future or dwelling on the past, mindfulness switches your focus to what's happening right now, enabling you to be fully engaged in the present moment.

Meditations that cultivate mindfulness have long been used to reduce stress, anxiety, depression, and other negative emotions. Some of these practices bring you into the present by focusing your attention on a single repetitive action, such as your breathing or a few repeated words. Other forms of mindfulness meditation encourage you to follow and then release internal thoughts or sensations. Mindfulness can also be applied to activities such as walking, exercising, or eating.

Using mindfulness to stay focused on the present might seem straightforward, but it takes practice to reap all the benefits. When you first start practicing, you'll likely find that your focus keeps wandering back to your worries or regrets. But don't get disheartened. Each time you draw your focus back to the present, you're strengthening a new mental habit that can help you break free of fretting about the past or stressing about the future. Using an app or audio download can also help focus your attention, especially when you're starting out.

A basic mindfulness meditation:

1. Find a quiet place where you won't be interrupted or distracted.

2. Sit on a comfortable chair with your back straight.

3. Close your eyes and find a point of focus, such as your breathing—the

sensation of air flowing into your nostrils and out of your mouth or your belly rising and falling—or a meaningful word that you repeat throughout the meditation.

4. Don't worry about distracting thoughts that go through your mind or about how well you're doing. If thoughts intrude your relaxation session, don't fight them, just gently turn your attention back to your point of focus, without judgment.

Rhythmic Movement And Mindful Exercise

The idea of exercising may not sound particularly soothing, but rhythmic exercise that gets you into a flow of repetitive movement can produce the relaxation response. Examples include:

• Running

• Walking

• Swimming

• Dancing

• Rowing

• Climbing

For Maximum Stress Relief, Add Mindfulness To Your Workout

While simply engaging in rhythmic exercise will help you relieve stress, adding a mindfulness component can benefit you even more.

As with meditation, mindful exercise requires being fully engaged in the present moment, paying attention to how your body feels right now, rather than your daily worries or concerns. Instead of zoning out or staring at a TV as you exercise, focus on the sensations in your limbs and how your breathing complements your movement.

If you're walking or running, for example, focus on the sensation of your feet touching the ground, the rhythm of your breath, and the feeling of the wind against your face. If you're resistance training, focus on coordinating your breathing with your movements and pay attention to how your body feels as you raise and lower the weights. And when your mind wanders to other thoughts, gently return your focus to your breathing and movement.

Yoga and Tai Chi

Yoga involves a series of both moving and stationary poses, combined with deep breathing. As well as reducing anxiety and stress, yoga can also improve flexibility, strength, balance, and stamina. Since injuries can happen when yoga is practiced incorrectly, it's best to learn by attending group classes, hiring a private teacher, or at least following video instructions. Once you've learned the basics, you can practice alone or with others, tailoring your practice as you see fit.

What type of yoga is best for stress?

Although almost all yoga classes end in a relaxation pose, classes that emphasize slow, steady movement, deep breathing, and gentle stretching are best for stress relief.

• Satyananda is a traditional form of yoga. It features gentle poses, deep relaxation, and meditation, making it suitable for beginners as well as anyone aiming primarily for stress reduction.

• Hatha yoga is also a reasonably gentle way to relieve stress and is suitable for beginners. Alternately, look for labels like gentle, for stress relief, or for beginners when selecting a yoga class.

• Power yoga, with its intense poses and focus on fitness, is better suited to those looking for stimulation as well as relaxation.

If you're unsure whether a specific yoga class is appropriate for stress relief, call the studio or ask the teacher.

Tai chi

If you've seen a group of people in the park slowly moving in sync, you've likely witnessed tai chi. Tai chi is a self-paced series of slow, flowing body movements. By focusing your mind on the movements and your breathing, you keep your attention on the present, which clears the mind and leads to a relaxed state.

173

Tai chi is a safe, low-impact option for people of all ages and fitness levels, including older adults and those recovering from injuries. As with yoga, it's best learned in a class or from a private instructor. Once you've learned the basics, you can practice alone or with others.

Tips For Starting A Relaxation Practice

Learning the basics of these relaxation techniques isn't difficult, but it takes regular practice to truly harness their stress-relieving power. Try setting aside at least 10 to 20 minutes a day for your relaxation practice.

Set aside time in your daily schedule. If possible, schedule a set time once or twice a day for your practice. If your schedule is already packed, try meditating while commuting on the bus or train, taking a yoga or tai chi break at lunchtime, or practicing mindful walking while exercising your dog.

Make use of smartphone apps and other aids. Many people find that smartphone apps or audio downloads can be useful in guiding them through different relaxation practices, establishing a regular routine, and keeping track of progress.

Expect ups and downs. Sometimes it can take time and practice to start reaping the full rewards of relaxation techniques such as meditation. The more you stick with it, the sooner the results will come. If you skip a few days or even a few weeks, don't get discouraged. Just start again and slowly build up to your old momentum.

Chapter 19: Pedal The Stress Away

Do you remember how happy you were riding your bicycle when you were young?

I remember my experience and I could give anything to feel the same way again; exciting, happy and a sense of unbridled freedom. It was just a great time without a care in the world.

Well, you do not have to look back to your childhood with such nostalgia because you can readily bring back those feel good moments you had on your bicycle then to the present to replace all the anxiety and worries you are facing now!

Don't you want to?

Cycling is another form of aerobic exercise which is great for stress relief, fitness and general well being. When you are overwhelmed by life's pressures simply hop on a bike and start pedaling for stress relief.

Being on the bike will take your mind off the problems that are bothering you, pump some feel good chemicals into your blood stream, pace you heart to leave you feeling refreshed and emotionally elated.

You can cycle after work, on weekends or your day off or even to work and while doing this, employ the meditative technique of mantra by chanting a positive phrase or word to the rhythm of your pedaling. I assure you that you will be surprised at how fats your mind will be cleared of the negativity and stress that you are facing.

Cycling is not an expensive endeavor, just buy a bicycle and you may start. It is not a vigorous if done for leisure or exercise and can be taken up by people of all ages.

Cycling will keep you fit, work out your heart for better health and emotional balance. It helps with the management of chronic conditions like diabetes, cardio vascular problems and high blood pressure.

The healthier and better you feel the less likely you are to be stressed. Get on your bike and enjoy the stress relieving benefits you have been missing.

Reading For Stress Relief

Reading is cathartic and is a great reliever of stress for people who are facing everyday pressures and adversity by relaxing the brain and managing the thought process.

When you read your mind travels away from the pressures you are facing; you sink into the story where you will find yourself in far away worlds. In the duration of your reading, you shall be transported away from your troubles and this helps to balance your emotional wellbeing.

Reading is a great mental exercise which stimulates brain activity thereby improving mental concentration and alertness. Stress fighting chemicals that give you a happy feeling are released into the brain. An active mind is strong and more likely to cope with daily pressures.

You will also fight stress from the motivation and hope you derive from reading biographies and motivational books. Books and other literature are sources of information which enables you to learn more and aid in problems solving.

A book will divert your thoughts from the lingering problems or worries that are stressing you out. Set aside a few hours in your day to read and you will experience how fulfilling it can be in your efforts at dealing with stress.

When you clear your mind of negativity even for a few hours, you will make huge strides in mental relaxation. With a relaxed mind you should be able to be more creative and relaxed enabling you to cope with stress. An active mind also slows down the aging process leaving you feeling younger physically and mentally; a strong healthy body is less prone to stress.

If the last time you read was for an exam or for a school assignment; make a hot cup of tea, make yourself comfortable on your favorite seat and immerse yourself into a book. The benefits for your life and health are great, you need to try it.

Get literature that appeals to you, a book, magazine or newspaper and make it a habit to read regularly for a less stress life every day.

Chapter 20: Move It Or Lose It

Often times with stress, we put ourselves in situations in which high levels of stress are a likely outcome. We put ourselves in such an expectative mindset that we do not realize that many causes of our stress are entirely avoidable. On average, people are awake for about 15-16 hours a day. During this period, there are many times in which we encounter stressful situations. When we encounter a stressful situation, you have to make a choice on how you are going to handle it. What are you going to do?

The first type of everyday situation we will analyze are basic social situations. These include interactions like ordering drive-thru food at a fast food restaurant, or telling the taxi driver where you want to go. While situations such as these can see monotonous, they are in fact important to your well being.

Stress and happiness are tied especially closely together in today's society. With the added freedoms and liberties in the world today, we are also given a choice unbeknownst to us that enables us to control the level of stress we have to put up with each day. Most people try to fit more into their day than they have time for. Usually, having too much in your schedule is a disaster waiting to happen for the said person. Someone who piles up high levels of tasks and responsibilities will end up in unhealthy social situations, fall into bad eating habits, and develop many other of the symptoms caused by prolonged levels of high stress.

In order for someone to lead a healthy life, that person must understand what needs to be done for that to happen. This person has to mentally commit to the fact that they will be able to lead a healthy and low-stress life. Unfortunately, when a person does not care to manage their schedule, it is almost inevitable that fast food and unhealthy junk will fall into that person's diet. Although people are always aware of all the sugar and junk they are ingesting, junk food is always easier to obtain than a fresh, healthy meal.

For all working people, it is sometimes the only option to go to the drive thru at McDonalds or Arby's. Having a fresh salad or soup is usually not even an option. Without properly caring to manage one's dietary schedule, junk food will become apart of everyday life, and will become detrimental. For example, my grandfather was what could be called a junk food addict. He was a fit, healthy man, but every day at his lunch break, he went to the local McDonalds for lunch. In fact, he went there so routinely, he was known by a first name basis. A few months before I was born, my grandfather passed away. He was only about 65, and he was in good shape. From what I know, he died due to a very poor diet, and he had been struggling with diet problems for years. I cannot begin to imagine the amount of stress he had to deal with everyday knowing that his work schedule was slowly killing him from the inside out.

When it comes to the actual task of planning an eating schedule, many people believe they know what is best for their bodies right off the bat. The thing is, people often forget to account that they want to have lives outside of work and eating. When executing a true, "healthy" eating schedule, it takes time and effort to complete. It is no longer acceptable to go to the McDonalds drive thru every day, or enjoy a Burger King Milkshake. It must be understood that to effectively reduce your dietary and lifestyle stress, a healthy diet must be incorporated.

Something that also must be understood is the "60 Minute Rule." A person should devote 60 complete hours a week to work, errands, responsibilities, and any other mandated functions. However, most people do not follow this rule. Instead of cleanly dividing the lines between their work and personal time, the two become mixed together. An errand might be put off and completed on a Saturday, or you might decide to go shopping in the middle of completing a project for work. Applying this careless philosophy to life can and will be detrimental to your health, as well as increase stress.

The brain functions best when it can deal with one activity or group of activities at a time. When work and personal time are mixed together, the mind and body can become exhausted fairly quickly. This is due to the fact that so many different hormones and parts of the brain are functioning at once and switching off constantly, exhaustion is the only thing that will ensue. The best way to avoid this, as we previously discussed, is to divide up your schedule into work and play, while doing your best to avoid overlapping between serious and personal matters.

Another good fact to know is that a person must live a well-rounded life in order to be fully happy. The way today's society has developed, this has become near impossible without prior planning. The professional jobs of today are now more demanding than they ever were, for a variety of reasons. The influx of new technology and the demand of the modern day workplace puts employees in positions in which it is expected that a 5 day work week is to be dedicated, along with select time on the weekends.

While this is unfortunate, it is still possible to lead a low stress, active lifestyle. While working and having a job is extremely important to owning a place to live, covering living expenses, and basically every necessity of life, having time for personal matters is also very important. Being able to do activities that you enjoy, whatever they may be, are very important in leading a low stress, while productive, professional lifestyle. Meeting up with friends, going out to a museum, or even relaxing in your own home can all be solutions to the monotony of everyday life.

When people attempt to cram as much as possible into their free days, even when these activities are intended to be fun and relaxing, can actually do the opposite. Stress ensues on a person when he or she is overwhelmed or feels pressured by a certain task. While waking up at 4 am to go on a nature hike and then immediately afterwards going out to a play with your friends before running back home to make dinner for a loved one can be nice for some people, for the majority, this is an example of a stressful schedule. One of the most common mistakes individuals make is attempting to cram in so many "relaxing" activities that they only become more stressed and exhausted. If someone continually tries to cram their days to do as much as possible, they lose time to truly spend with friends and family, and actually due activities that they look forward to and enjoy.

Stress is a natural factor in every professional's and individual's life. However, a poor diet and large amounts of ill-advised activities can lead to a large increase in the stress you suffer every day.

While there are many causes, stress in many cases can be caused by the individual him/herself overloading their everyday schedule. This leads to unhealthy exhaustion, and a feeling of emptiness that you did not truly get the most out of the day that you desired. In fact, many people forget about their health, diet, and personal well being when living busy, cluttered lives. Living a high activity lifestyle is only acceptable when it is acknowledged, and it is made clear that time is set aside for true fun and relaxation.

Conclusions

The stress prevention techniques within this book can give you the certainty, confidence and conviction to take control of your stressful situations so that you can prevent stress, using fun and easy to apply stress prevention techniques. We have looked at the way top achievers prevent stress and how you can understand the causes, the effects and symptoms of stress. We looked at the consequences of you taking action ...or not, in relation to stress. We have looked at control, security and acceptance and some of the main causes of stress and how the CSA can affect or be the reason behind these things. We looked at anchoring, we looked at the use of "your book", and we considered the twenty one day rule using simple and "easy to do" things that every day in a small way, can help to make you happier and more stress free.

You have read about looking into people who have great relaxation and stress prevention stress methods that you could possibly model. We have also recorded and practiced the closed eye relaxation process that with time can be a superb daily routine to keep you on top of your game.

I hope you took great benefits from the closed eye relaxation exercise and that you listened to your recording over and over again to make sure it becomes a habit for you. Stress prevention can be achieved and you deserve it. You do deserve to be stress free and I look forward to hearing how you have used these techniques to create more energy and well-being for yourself.

CPSIA information can be obtained
at www.ICGtesting.com
Printed in the USA
BVHW050844020622
638737BV00014B/291